»You just do it.
You force yourself to get up.
You force yourself to
put one foot in front of the other,
and God damn it,
you refuse to let it get to you.
You fight. You cry. You curse.
Then you go about the
business of living.
That's how I've done it.
There is no other way.«

ELIZABETH TAYLOR

D1637611

e.

EHRLIN PUBLISHING

Perimenopower – The Ultimate Guide Through The Change

Original Swedish title: Perimenopower – hitta din superkraft när hormonerna svänger
Translated to English by Karin Shearman

© 2018 Katarina Wilk and Ehrlin Publishing AB
Photo of author: Johan Strindberg
Graphic Design: Eva Lindeberg
ISBN: 978-91-88375-38-4
www.ehrlinpublishing.com

KATARINA WILK

PERI MENO POWER

The Ultimate Guide Through the Change

Translated by Karin Shearman

e.

EHRLIN PUBLISHING

Contents

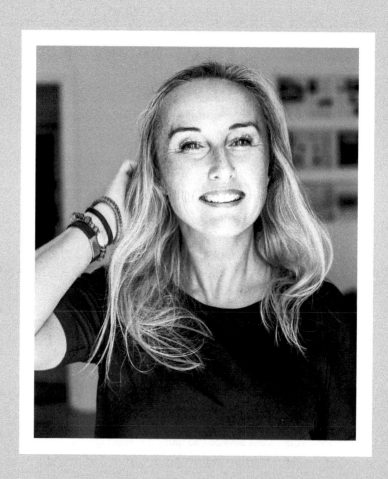

Foreword

A few years ago, things started happening to my body that I did not recognize. I couldn't sleep, had panic attacks and sudden bouts of sweating. There were so many odd things happening all at once and I felt sad and confused. Perhaps the way you feel right now? Worried, low and sad? Like all you want is to get rid of this strange condition, although you can barely explain what it is.

During a girls' dinner party, when I reluctantly admitted how I felt, everyone started laughing. In the end, we all laughed so hard that we cried. *Everyone* had similar symptoms, but none of us realized at the time that it could be because we were getting close to the time when our periods would stop. We still had regular bleedings and we were only in our forties. We had heard that you could experience similar things during the menopause, but surely that was something that happened when you were getting close to or past the age of 50?

Naturally a curious person, I decided to find out more. When I realized how little collective knowledge there is about this subject, and how many theories and advice were floating around, I made the decision to write this book.

My whole working life has been spent as a writer and editor with a focus towards health, training, and medicine. I have always had a great interest in the female body as I am fascinated by how amazing it is. For example, that a woman can carry and give birth to babies is incredible. Your body is a miracle and you need to look after it carefully, especially during sensitive periods such as puberty, pregnancy, and perimenopause – times when your female sex hormones go crazy.

This book will not replace professional health care by licensed doctors; if you feel really unwell you need to get help. I won't be saying that estrogen is better than natural medicines or that cardio training is better than strength training. Instead, I will present different alternatives and solutions, and give you the option of making an informed decision. I am offering you a chance to take charge of your life and I hope you will realize that you don't have to live with these symptoms if you don't want to, as there are things you can do to feel better.

The one thing I can promise you is that I have tried everything to feel better and today I am in better physical and mental shape than ever. But it has been a long and winding road, and it is this road that I want to share with you. There is such a lack of knowledge on this subject, but I hope that this book will help to change this. A tip I can give you straight away is to stop googling your symptoms. Most of them are conveniently compiled here for you.

Between you and me, most of my friends are »patients« of mine. I am known in my group of girls as the one who pretends to be a doctor. At the first sign of a symptom, I try to help them the best I can and with the knowledge I have. Even if it's just to support them there and then. I want to help you too. I want you to feel more secure after reading this book. That you will understand more about what is going on inside your body and that you will know how to turn the negatives into positives. This period in your life isn't an illness, it's a phase. A phase that affects most women in the world.

I want to make you feel that you are not alone, but also give you the knowledge of what happens in the female body. For example, did you know that what happens in your body before your last period can go on for as long as 10–15 years before your periods end? Most of the symptoms you have are not unusual and they are the result of your hormones being completely off track.

This book is in two parts. The first part is based upon my own experiences which you may recognize in yourself. To make it easier for you, I will guide you through the necessary terms and describe what happens inside your body. The second part is about what you can do in order to feel the best you can. My hope is that you will use this book as a guide on your journey to find your superpower when the hormones swing.

This is a book for those of you who are 35 and older and interested in the reasons for why you are sleepless, sweaty, and down, and want to get the best tips for waking up well-rested, fresh, and happy. I want to help you find yourself again. You could say that this book is the result of extremely difficult hormonal storms in combination with a somewhat obsessive interest in medicine and a curiosity that irritates some and fascinates others. All medical facts have been checked by Evelina Sande Idenfeldt who is a senior doctor of gynecology and obstetrics and who runs a women's clinic in Sweden.

Perimenopower is a new word, invented by me. It comes from the word *perimenopause*, which is the term for the time before your last period, and *power*. To be a woman is, in itself, a superpower and perimenopower is exactly what you need to get through this difficult phase. This power is already inside of you but, with all of these strange symptoms, it disappears out of sight. Even if it may not feel like it at the moment, you are incredibly strong. How many times didn't things happen in your life and all you wanted to do was to curl up in a little ball? You may have done just that for a while, but you always manage to get up again. Use that strength now. Your perimenopower is there, I promise.

Camilla D

Part 1

PERIMENOPAUSE

Just Hit Me!

»If I don't sleep soon
I'm going to die in one
way or another.«

A TEXT MESSAGE TO MY SISTER A FEW YEARS BACK

The CHAPTER 1

My Story

My first symptoms began soon after I turned 40. Because I didn't know where to turn, or even if my symptoms were anything to be taken seriously, I started to look for answers wherever I could find them. The questions were numerous, and so difficult to find answers to since I could hardly explain the symptoms even to myself. Why did I feel so low? Why was I unable to sleep? Why did I wake at night with palpitations and sheets drenched in sweat?

I'm not depressed – I just want to sleep

I remember it vividly. It was just before Christmas and I simply could not get to sleep. It wasn't that I had difficulties going to sleep or that I woke up several times in the night. I simply didn't sleep a wink, not even one second throughout the night. Have you ever experienced this? Then you know that the only thing you think about when you can't sleep is how much you want to sleep, which builds up panic and frustration that doesn't make falling asleep any easier.

I explained away the sleeplessness as stress. You know, as can happen around Christmas. There is food to be cooked, presents to be bought, and trips to grandparents and in-laws to be planned. No wonder, you have a thousand things on your mind. But no matter how hard I tried, I couldn't shut my brain down, so I went to my doctor.

The doctor asked if I was finding things difficult at the

moment. If I was feeling low. I had to stop myself from shoving the stethoscope down her throat. Of course I felt low, most people who get no sleep feel low. It was a badly formulated question. But I was starting to panic. I felt so bad and I was getting no help. And I simply couldn't get to sleep.

A day or two later, I returned to the medical center and started to cry out of hopelessness. The doctor realized that this person had to sleep or something terrible would happen. So, she prescribed some strong sleeping tablets.

– Depression or exhaustion, she said, and despite feeling neither depressed nor exhausted, I nodded while sobbing. I had no other alternative.

I took one of the strong sleeping pills that same evening. But it was the first, and definitely the last, time I tried that. I suffered terrible hallucinations, and what should have been a beauty sleep ended with me hardly daring to go to sleep again. The nightmares I had that night were worse than all horror films put together. So much blood, so many babies without heads. When I woke, I was completely wiped out and filled with such anxiety that I thought I may need admitting to a psychiatric unit. So, although I'd been asleep, it was a sleep I could have done without. I remember my next visit to the medical center when I told the doctor about my night filled with nightmares.

– I think you should start a course of anti-depressants, you

INSOMNIA

Insomnia is the medical term for sleeplessness. It means that you are unable to sleep, you sleep badly, or wake early. It can be temporary or more permanent.

Where did this
unease come from?
Sometimes I awoke from
paranoid nightmares.
Completely soaked,
with a racing pulse.

show all the signs of being depressed, said the doctor.

– I don't want to take anti-depressants. I'm not depressed, I just want to sleep. It must be something else.

– It's probably just temporary, continue with the sleeping tablets and you'll be fine. These things just happen sometimes.

I was terribly sad when I left. My questions about why I felt the way I did had not been answered, instead it felt as though the doctor had tried to persuade me that I was depressed even though I didn't feel like that at all. I felt more confused when I left than when I had arrived. Have you ever experienced this – leaving the doctor and wondering if you'd even been helped?

Seeing connections and looking for solutions

Once Christmas was over, we went to Spain. I was feeling panicked, since I still didn't know why my body refused to sleep. The panic grew every day as I got more and more tired. I simply could not get to sleep. But since I had lived in France during my youth, I knew that you could get strong medicines over the counter in southern Europe, and I was not disappointed. The local pharmacist in the Andalusian mountain village recommended a supplement of melatonin, a natural sleep hormone produced by the body but decreases with age. Melatonin is sold as a supplement in Europe and the US but not in Sweden. I had taken it a few years earlier for sleeping problems caused by jetlag when I was in the US and it had worked then.

I took melatonin and finally I could begin to sleep a little again. But I still wondered what was going on, my brain was working overtime. What caused the sleeplessness? I had also started to suffer from low blood sugar more often and had to eat regularly in order not to feel weak and shaky. I had never experienced it so vividly before. Have you experienced problems with blood sugar? Then you will know how weak and faint you can suddenly feel. Like you just want to devour an entire bar of chocolate just to get some energy back.

Then I suddenly realized that during the past fall I had also suffered panic attacks and sometimes felt a pressure across my chest. As if my body was constantly tense and I couldn't relax. I had never felt this before, it was completely new to me. Where did this unease come from? Sometimes I awoke from paranoid nightmares. Completely soaked, with a racing pulse. I felt seriously ill and worried. Has this happened to you too?

I refused to accept the doctor's theories of exhaustion and depression and I wanted to see if there could be any solutions to my problems, other than sleeping pills and anti-depressants. I was going to try to find a solution myself, or at least find out what options there were to help me, and if it worked for me perhaps I could then help others.

Having said that, I once again want to clarify that what you are going through isn't an illness but a phase that most women go through. Some of us suffer more, others less, and sometimes it's hard to say which came first, the chicken or the egg. Do you get anxious from not sleeping or do you not sleep because you are anxious? In the end, it doesn't really matter. You need to take what you are experiencing seriously, and not just accept living with symptoms that can be cured relatively easily.

PERIMENOPAUSE

The time before your final period.
A period in your life when you are
experiencing hormonal changes. It
can start as early as age 35, but for
many the age is between 40 and 45.

Eventually I discovered tricks that reduced all my symptoms, such as sweating, feeling low, and sleeplessness. This is what I want to share with you throughout the rest of the book.

CHAPTER 2

You are not alone

I have always been fascinated by how the body works. The fact that it works as well as it does is incredible. So many things have to click, and most of the time they actually do – we are usually in pretty good shape. Therefore, it can be even harder once you realize that your body no longer works perfectly. That was how I felt, anyhow. I am not a hypochondriac and I have rarely been ill, so when my body began to go on strike and strange symptoms appeared both in body and mind, it felt very strange. What is going on? Why do I feel so peculiar? No one had warned me about unexplainable symptoms that appear from nowhere.

We are all in the same boat

I started to read online, in books, in research papers. I watched every TV interview I could find, plowed through podcasts in search of the slightest recognition. What I realized early on was that I was entering something that simply wasn't spoken about. Not with your friends, your husband, or even your doctor. You are not supposed to talk about sweaty nights, insomnia, or panic attacks.

Why is it tabu?

If you ask your mother, she will most likely say that she never had any problems at all. Or that she doesn't remember. Not even the older generation wants to talk about it, maybe

»When I had my first
hot flush at night and
googled night sweats,
I was terrified.
Then I told my boss
and she just laughed
in recognition.«

LINN, 43

them least of all. My theory is that it's either taboo, in other words too personal to talk about, or that you don't connect the symptoms with hormone changes when they might come as early as at 35–40 years of age.

With a little luck, you have a mother who remembers how it was for her and supports you through it. These problems can be hereditary. If your mother had problems, you may have similar ones. If she only had difficulty in sleeping and nothing else, it's plausible that you too will only suffer from sleep issues.

My mother can't remember having any discomforts at all. Perhaps she belongs to the group of mothers who doesn't want to talk about these things and, naturally, this must be respected. But do ask your mother if you get the chance. It can give you a hint of what is to come, and the chances are that she has valuable tips and hints about what worked for her. Keep in mind, though, that she belongs to a different generation which means that she may have opinions that you don't agree with, things that may have changed culturally or evidentially since she had her most unstable period.

But do remember, there is nothing wrong with you. Don't think that you have been hit by a dangerous disease, something that's not normal. Most of it is probably completely in order.

Now that I have started talking about my problems and written a book about the perimenopause, most of my friends admit to having symptoms. They range from my little sister, who has just turned 42, telling me that she feels a bit low during certain periods (without obvious reason), to my colleague who is 37 and cannot sleep. My perception was that, earlier on, talking about the subject with girlfriends was like walking on thin ice, but I promise you – our dinners are more fun now than ever. I also feel closer to the women at work since we started talking about the strange things we had been experiencing. A close friend of mine, for example, told me how she had been dating a new man and how he asked her in the middle of the night whether she wanted some medicine to relieve her fever. What do you think her date would have thought if she'd told the truth?

It's not a disease!

– I didn't have a fever last night, I am just entering the menopause.

Several times, after these dinners, my stomach aches from too much laughter. Try bringing up the subject with your friends, the chances are that you will laugh and cry at the same time at everyone's stories. You will also become closer to them if you just dare to start talking about it.

Hard to see the whole picture

The feeling I had when I went to the doctor, as I described in the previous chapter, was that no one was listening to me. They thought they knew what was going on in my body, but I knew they were talking nonsense. I don't know if it comes down to a lack of knowledge or if they don't believe the symptoms even exist. But they very much do.

Of course, it can sometimes be difficult to see that the symptoms are connected when, separately, they can have many different reasons, and in small doses they might not even be seen as abnormal or strange. But I wish that the connection between these symptoms and hormonal changes could be made in the medical center before they prescribe sleeping pills and anti-depressants. They should ask you about your menstrual cycle instead of assuming that you are suffering from exhaustion. They should ask about your sleep, if you have anxiety or hot flushes at night. And when they have managed to understand what is going on in your body, the first step should be to refer you to a gynecologist who is a specialist in the female hormone-filled body.

Some gynecologists want to measure your hormone levels, while others understand about your hormone changes by looking at your symptoms. Once I put two and two together and visited my gynecologist, it was like a weight being lifted off my shoulders. She looked at me and smiled and said that she would sort me out. This was the first time I heard that my symptoms had something to do with the menopause. That hormones can change for a long time before your periods stop. One of the positives was that I had been seeing her for several years. She had followed me from pregnancy to peri-menopause. It was a great relief to talk to someone with the experience and the ability to put words to these things that I had never experienced before.

Demand the right kind of care!

She asked me to keep a diary of my symptoms. I began taking notes every day when I experienced something strange that could be related to this. By doing so she could determine that it really was hormonal and make me understand that it was linked to my menstrual cycle and nothing else. I have an awful lot to thank this woman for.

Having a gynecologist who you want to go back to and who knows your history is something that I wish all women had. It really helps in this jumble of symptoms. Ask your gynecologist to explain to you in a simple-to-understand way. Perhaps you lack the energy or simply don't want to absorb everything in as much detail as I do, with my obsessive interest in anything to do with the body. But try to understand the basics. It will make things a lot easier for you. I will do my best to explain, and, for you to get the whole picture, in the next chapter I will clarify some terms.

She asked me to
keep a diary of my
symptoms. I began taking
notes every day when I
experienced something
strange that could be
related to this.

»What do you mean, the menopause? I had just turned 38, had no children and was suddenly having daily panic attacks. I was completely convinced that I was very ill.«

ANNA, 38

CHAPTER 3

Through terminology

What enters your mind when you hear the term menopause? Apart from finding it to be a negatively charged term, to many it is also surrounded in confusion. If you ask your female friends what it means, most will probably say it is when your periods end at around the age of 50. If you ask how long this period lasts, most will have no clue. A maximum of a couple of years is what most people think, and the majority believe that the menopause is the beginning of the end. Perhaps you don't want to realize when you are 35–40 years old that the symptoms you are experiencing are related to hormones and aging. That would mean you are starting to get old.

We fear getting old – that can't be denied. Who wants to get old, really? Personally, I would like to have stayed 35 for the rest of my life. But getting older is inevitable and I think it's time that we start to see the power in aging. I believe it may be our own fault that the term *menopause* is so negatively charged. Age doesn't have to be something unattractive. Have you, for example, seen Elon Musk's mother? Maye Musk still works as a supermodel at 69 years of age. Google her and you will see. She is in fact one of the most beautiful women I've seen.

Fear of getting old?

The menopause is a point in time

Not many people in their mid-30s think that the symptoms they are experiencing are to do with hormones. In the same way, it is often difficult for doctors to figure it out. Instead, you are looking for other diagnoses because you don't have knowledge about hormonal problems or how much of a woman's life is affected by them.

If you look up the word menopause online, you might get confused. In Sweden we use the word climacteric for the menopausal transition. Plus a lot of other words so it's quite confusing. But actually we are not the only ones that are confused. The International Menopause Society (IMS) that has members in 62 countries, stated already 1999 that there was a misuse of terminology related to this field which which was confusing among healthcare providers, media, and the public. There was a question if to keep the word climacteric in the medical lexicon or not. They did eventually keep the word, but it's not used that much anymore. Instead the words perimenopause, menopause and postmenopause are used for the transition in a womans life.

When you delve deeper into what the different words mean, you find that that they have sometimes mixed up the terms. First and foremost, the climacteric and the menopause are *not* the same thing. The climacteric has to do with the transition – the perimenopause. The climacteric isn't a point in time but a *period.* The menopause isn't a period but a *point in time.*

The climacteric isn't a point in time, but a **PERIOD**.
The menopause isn't a period, but a **POINT IN TIME**.

When you have not had your period for 12 consecutive months, you are said to have reached the menopause, the time when your periods have stopped completely. The period *before* you stop having monthly periods is called the change or the perimenopause. But on the internet and in various books, articles, and podcasts another term exists, the *premenopause*, making it even more confusing. So, if the change is the perimenopause, what is the premenopause? The time period before the perimenopause? An early stage of the perimenopause? Why even talk about various stages of a stage that happens before something that's yet to come? Well, you hear how confusing it is …

I have made it easy for myself and I'm going to make it easy for you too. For the sake of simplicity, I will use only two terms, and these are the only ones you need to bear in mind when you read this book. These are **PERIMENOPAUSE** and **MENOPAUSE**. Perimenopause = before your periods stop. Menopause = when they do stop. Forget the terms the pre-menopause and the climacteric.

To become a dab hand in what the perimenopause and menopause are all about, I will explain everything I know – »Doctor« Wilk at your service.

Perimenopause – the hormonal worry starts

As I said, the perimenopause is the period before your periods stop. This is the period that this book really is about, and how to tackle the hormonal changes and the symptoms that often come with it.

There is no universal age for when the hormones start

changing, but normally the symptoms are experienced the most between the ages of 40 and 50. They can come as early as right after 35. We are all different, but for most people, they can go on for several years. The purpose of this book is to help you through the perimenopause regardless of you entering it two or fifteen years before your periods stop. I want you to remember the word perimenopause. I want you to use it when you go to your doctor. I don't want you to google it. Promise me that you will stop googling. I want you to tell your doctor or gynecologist that you believe you have entered the perimenopause and that you need help to tackle it.

> **PERIMENOPAUSE** Comes from the Greek where peri means *around*. In other words, the word peri + menopause means: the time around the menopause. This is the period where you will notice the biggest changes.

Menopause – when your periods have stopped completely

The next term to bear in mind is *menopause*. It may not come as a complete surprise, but we will all have one last period. The menopause occurs when you have gone 12 months since your last period. Then you are on the other side. On that side, you don't need to think about sanitary towels or contraceptives. It's the period-free side where you can no longer bear children.

Some people find it difficult when the periods stop, while others are elated. Some slip into existential depression and, of course, in a way this is a passage in life that makes you think. Regardless of whether you have been able to have children earlier, the menopause is a sign that it's now definitely over, you have no more chances to produce a biological offspring. I understand why this makes many people feel low, for after all, childbirth is probably among the greatest things that can happen in one's life – but at the same time, think about all the other things life can offer. So, don't despair if you find it difficult to handle the changes you are facing. We will sort this out.

> **MENOPAUSE** Comes from the French word *menèspausie* (which derives from Latin) where *menès* means monthly and *pausie* means to end. The term menopause is, in other words, an ending of something that happens every month. The menopause occurs when you have not had a period for 12 months.

CHAPTER 4

What's wrong with our bodies?

The body is one big mystery. Just think about it, we all start our lives in our mother's belly. We, in turn, carry our children inside of us. The fact that the development from a tiny egg to a small human normally progresses well is nothing short of a miracle. The fact that it normally stays that way and that you stay healthy through the greater part of your life is, in many ways, also a miracle.

Meet the hormones estrogen and progesterone

Many things in our bodies affect our well-being, and something central to our health are hormones. They affect metabolism, reproduction, sexual maturity, libido, and many other things. The hormonal system is made up of something known as endocrine glands. These glands produce hormones. They are transported via your blood like small armies with specific goals.

These hormones have many special skills. Some are experts at reducing stress, others make sure your body grows and develops the way it's programmed to do. One thing's for sure, the hormones are very determined and highly skilled at their job. Just like people who are experts in their field of work, hormones know exactly what they are supposed to do.

»I would do anything
to feel like myself again.
It's not reasonable to feel
this way for such a
long time.«

LISA, 43

A well-known hormone that has gained superstar status in the world of health is *insulin*. Insulin wins first prize when it comes to lowering your blood sugar level. After devouring a packet of sweets, insulin works hard to take care of that sugar for you.

However, the hormones that are your best friends – and sometimes your worst enemy, which we will return to later – are the female sex hormones, *estrogen* and *progesterone*. They are sometimes known as ovarian hormones since they have their headquarters in your ovaries. They are the ones that ensure you have your period every month and that your body can develop a baby should you be fertilized.

But as with any best friend, there may be a time when the two of you don't completely agree, and even though estrogen and progesterone normally work *for* you, suddenly they may start causing trouble. The time when your hormone levels start changing is the time you could say you have entered the perimenopause. Your hormones start acting like unruly teenagers going bananas, leaving you completely unable to predict what they will do next.

The reason you feel unwell during this period is that the level of sex hormones changes. There is unease in the hormone camp. You could liken the swinging hormones to a dance. When you are feeling well it's largely thanks to your hormones. When you are feeling ill it's also often because of your hormones. Your sex hormones dance around in your body and their relationship with each other affects your entire being.

Do you remember the movie *Dirty Dancing*? It's not until the main characters are completely in phase with each other that they are able to complete the lift at the end. For you to be best able to help your body, it's good to understand that what happens between your hormones affects your whole well-being. Which is exactly what happens between the characters in *Dirty Dancing*; when they are in harmony, the dance goes well. When your hormones work together in harmony, you feel well.

So, now I would like to give you a better insight into how sex hormones work. I understand if you find it hard to grasp all of this but try to get as much insight as you need in order to better understand your body.

The basis of the menstrual cycle

In order to describe what happens to the hormones during the perimenopause, we need to look at a normal menstrual cycle. And without complicating matters more than needed, here follows a basic description of how the hormones work in a typical menstrual cycle.

Each menstrual cycle lasts on average 28 days. For some it's as short as 25 days and for others it can be longer. During a menstrual cycle, the levels of estrogen and progesterone vary. Some days the difference is greater, and this is what makes you notice an imbalance in your body, which can manifest itself physically or mentally.

The menstrual cycle runs from the first day of your period to the first day of your next period. In the beginning and the end of the cycle, your levels of both estrogen and progesterone are low. One week after your period starts, estrogen levels begin to rise, while progesterone levels remain at the same level a while longer. Approximately two weeks after your period, estrogen levels peak while progesterone levels are slowly gathering speed. After this, you are ovulating, during which your body is at its most fertile and you are ready to conceive. You could say that the ovulation in the middle of your menstrual cycle is like reaching climax. The progesterone reaches its top level and the estrogen starts to dip.

During the last week before your period, the levels of both estrogen and progesterone go down. Finally, you will have your period and your menstrual cycle will begin all over again. In other words, there is a substantial change in hormone levels while you still bleed regularly. But these changes are normal. They are the same every menstrual cycle.

When you enter the perimenopause, it doesn't work the same anymore; instead your hormones begin to act more like headless chickens, running around with no direction. They are no longer following each other like they used to, when the »hormone dance« worked as normal. All of a sudden, one is pulling away from the other uncontrollably while the other is fighting back and your body is starting to become very unsettled. Just like in the film, when they are not in sync, the dance doesn't work.

My gynecologist
always tells me that it's no
wonder I have problems
during the perimenopause
since I have also had
severe PMS.

Progesterone levels drop first

The first hormone to decrease during perimenopause is progesterone. Many of the symptoms that arise are caused by dipping progesterone levels. Or, to be more accurate, a reduced progesterone level in combination with a stable estrogen level. We are simply getting too little progesterone in relation to how much estrogen we have left. The »normal« changes that we have during our menstrual cycle are completely disrupted.

Hormone changes are natural, but when they start changing in a way that's unnatural in relation to each other, then hormone chaos ensues. During the perimenopause, one could say that the sex hormones refuse to work together in the way they have always done before. It may feel like they are acting unpredictably, and we must help them to find each other again. Because if your hormones find peace, so will you.

Severe PMS that never ends

Perhaps you have suffered from PMS at some time? PMS is an abbreviation for premenstrual syndrome and it usually occurs 1–7 days before your period, as a result of an imbalance in your hormones. Some women are more susceptible to the hormonal imbalance, thus experiencing PMS more than others.

PMS can manifest itself both physically and mentally. Do you have tender breasts before periods? This is typical of PMS. Or do you feel really low, crying at the slightest thing? This is also common with PMS. Many people liken the perimeno-

pause to severe PMS. Perimenopause differs from PMS in that
it feels as if it never ends. After all, PMS has a beginning and
an end, and normally limits itself to a maximum of one week
per month. The PMS-like problems can also be experienced
as more severe during the perimenopause.

You can also see similarities between the perimenopause
and other periods in life when your hormones are disrupted.
If you, for example, found it difficult going through puberty
and pregnancy, you run a greater risk of being affected
during the perimenopause as well. But if you danced your
way through these periods without major problems, you run a
smaller chance of having problems now.

My gynecologist always tells me that it's no wonder I have
problems during the perimenopause since I have also had
severe PMS. Some people are simply more sensitive to hormonal changes than others. What do you think is the case for
you? Do you remember your puberty? If so, you might see
similarities with what you are going through now, or predict
what lies ahead.

High sensitivity may have something to do with it

I also believe that you can find other causes that affect how
sensitive you are to hormonal unease. Some women tend to
be more sensitive to *everything* than others. Can you see a
pattern among your group of friends? Is there anyone who is
more sensitive and generally more affected by what's going on
around them than others?

Have you heard about HSP? It stands for *Highly Sensitive
Person* and means that a person has a »highly sensivtive perso-

nality,« that you experience things at a higher, or subtler, level than others. In other words, you have a more finely tuned system for picking up signals and sensory impressions that others might not notice. Imagine if, as an HSP, you sense your hormones more than others?

What is HSP?

I, myself, am a hormonally sensitive person and probably have a slight slant towards HSP. I have big feelings and take in everything that goes on around me. But during this period when I felt so unwell, I pulled myself together for the first time in a long while. I refused to accept that just because I am highly sensitive I would have a »breakdown« only from a bunch of strange symptoms.

I thought about my children, how hard it can be to watch your happy mum not being so happy any longer. I thought about my puberty when I felt really awful. For their sake and my own, I therefore tried to change my mindset. Of course, I still have times or days when I am not at my best, but overall, I feel better and better with age and I believe much of it is about attitude. A close friend of mine, who is a psychologist, often says that she thinks I have a strong resistance, that nowadays I can remain upright even in stormy weather.

What I am trying to say is, regardless of how sensitive you are to hormonal changes, I am convinced that you can improve your situation and work on your resistance, even if much of it is genetic. I believe I am a pretty good example of this and maybe you will be too if you try following my advice. I hope I'll be able to help you and that there are bits and pieces in the following chapters that will make you feel better.

CHAPTER 5

This can happen

By now, you know that the symptoms I am describing are due to the fact that the hormones are starting to change. This happens to most women but to different degrees. The amount of hormonal problems you experience can also depend upon where in the world you live. Factors like diet, lifestyle, and climate may affect us more than we think, and the symptoms may not just be dependent on our physiology, that is, how our bodies work.

Different symptoms in different parts of the world

PubMed is a database with over 26 million medical-related references to studies, which sometimes are used as a basis for wider research. It's like an enormous digital library covering the world's medical studies. In 2014, a major examination of the 64 most important studies in PubMed covering the symptoms apparent in perimenopause was conducted by a Polish team. The idea of this study was to examine how the symptoms during perimenopause differ in various parts of the world.

The results proved very interesting. In the US, aching joints and muscles were most common. Australian women suffered the most from vasomotor symptoms (including hot flushes and sweating) and sexual dysfunction. In Africa there was no clear pattern, instead several symptoms were prominent. In Europe, sleeping problems and depression weighed heaviest, and Asian women generally had milder symptoms than those in other parts of the world. The fact that there are geographical differences I find very interesting. Why do you think this is?

The Polish study did not reach any conclusion as to *why* the symptoms were different for different groups of women in the world, but it's probable that lifestyle has an influence. Food culture differs a great deal in the different parts of the world, and we also have different views on physical activity. An average Westerner may exercise at the gym for a couple of hours per week, while in other places in the world you may have to walk 10 kilometers per day to fetch water. My view is that lifestyle may be part of the explanation as to why there are such differences in which perimenopause symptoms appear in different parts of the world.

I also believe that the way we see ourselves differs around the world. In some parts, age is associated with authority while, in the West, we have a very deep-rooted youth culture where we do everything in our power not to grow old. »Growing old« is still seen as something negative, and this perception affects women more than men. Not least, this is apparent in the beauty industry which markets all sorts of potions and treatments aimed at making us look younger. In such a culture, it's no wonder that nearing the menopause is seen as the beginning of the end for us women.

When we discuss the menopause, I often get the feeling that it is from the position of a martyr. Some of us tend to complain about this and that, often combined with a wish for people to feel sorry for us. What if we could turn things around, and choose to see aging as something liberating instead? As the start of a new chapter in life that we actually should feel grateful to experience? Think about this when you are feeling low – is it you or the society you live in that makes you feel bad?

As I have mentioned earlier, your sleep is one of the most important things for you to feel well, but your self-image is equally important during this period. Society may have told you that you must stay young, but you are the one who can choose to embrace aging. Do as the Maya Indians: Despite the different discomforting symptoms, they looked forward to the menopause. It meant a sense of freedom and a higher status for them. Even in India, as early as the 1970s, this period in a woman's life was described as one which would give her new possibilities, like laughing and joking with men in public.

Although it's rather tragic that women did not reach the same status as men until they stopped having periods every month, it's an example of how the view of women in different countries is associated with the view of the menopause and how you experience your perimenopause. In the Western world, we are fed the image that we should be young and beautiful and that the menopause stops you from being so, while in some countries it's a symbol of new-won freedom. I think you should be grateful of your aging; many of us never get the chance to grow old. Just being alive is a gift. Don't ever forget that. Find your perimenopower and feel freer and more beautiful than ever. It's in your hands only!

What are we suffering from?

So, what is it really on this smorgasbord of perimenopause symptoms? Well, the list is never-ending and varies from woman to woman. But there are some symptoms that appear more frequently than others.

How about irregular periods, unusually heavy bleeding or spotting, sleeplessness, weight gain, hot flushes, palpitations, night sweats, mood swings, headaches, incontinence, dry mucus membranes, reduced sex drive, joint and muscle pain, tiredness, anxiety, depression, and panic attacks. Doesn't it make you sweaty just reading about it?

The first symptom is normally a change in your bleeding pattern, where your periods will become more frequent or infrequent than before.

In this book I want to help you to become well-rested, fresh, and alert. Then you will find the key to your super-power. Until then, I will go through some of the things that occur in your body when you are sleepless, sweaty, and down in the dumps.

Like having a bucket of warm juice poured over you

I will never forget the first time I was in a meeting and it felt

SYMPTOMS

irregular periods
unusually heavy bleeding
spotting
sleeplessness
weight gain
hot flushes
palpitations
night sweats
mood swings
headaches
frequent need to urinate
dry mucus membranes
reduced sex drive
joint and muscle pain
tiredness
anxiety
depression
panic attacks

Have you ever woken up
in the middle of the night
with sweat pouring down
your whole upper body and
hair and, to top it all off,
your sheets completely
soaked?

as though I was about to have a panic attack. First, a feeling of anxiety came over me and soon after that I had a feeling of warmth in my upper body and I began to have severe cold sweats. Have you ever woken up in the middle of the night with sweat pouring down your whole upper body and hair and, to top it all off, your sheets completely soaked? Then you know what I am talking about.

This has happened to me a few times and it's a very strange experience. To me, it happened mostly at night but sometimes also during the day. To begin with, it was mostly just before my period, but then it started happening whenever. Before I knew what it was, I feared that I had a serious illness. I can advise you not to google night sweats – all sorts of information will come up. I have said it before and I will say it again as a reminder, stop googling! It will only make you more confused. When my best friend told me that during her period she had something verging on bouts of fever once a month, I knew exactly what it was. It wasn't a fever, it was hot flushes!

Having hot flushes is quite normal during the perimenopause. It's estimated that 70–75 percent of all women experience hot flushes, and it's the most common symptom to try to get medical help for. During the perimenopause, hot flushes can appear for a while, only to suddenly disappear and come back later on.

As with everything else, there is no uniformity for everybody; instead, the frequency and degree are completely individual. For some women, the hot flushes don't appear until they are very near the menopause, for others they continue way after their last period.

A hot flush can range from a mild warm sensation in your body to the feeling that a bucket of warm juice has been poured over you. Warm, wet, and sticky, with a topping of something that feels like anxiety. The way most people describe the classic hot flush is the feeling of heat over your face, shoulders, head, and upper body. You often feel in advance that a hot flush is imminent. You can feel worried, anxious, or just have a feeling that something is wrong with your body.

What happens during a hot flush is that the body heats up, just like when you have a fever or exercise hard. A study with sensors has shown that the body's outer temperature can raise by up to four degrees during a hot flush. The blood flow rises which makes the skin hot and flushing. The body's reaction to this acute rise in temperature is to cool down. The same system that kicks in during a fever is triggered here too and for many women this means a feeling of having an attack of extreme sweating. Some start to shiver despite being sweaty and some don't sweat at all. And then there are the women who experience a hot sweat and a cold sweat at the same time.

Some women experience other vasomotor problems during this period (problems to do with the blood vessels' ability to expand and contract). It can be palpitations, irregular heartbeat, or a racing heart – it seems like anything and everything can occur during the perimenopause.

Personally, I suffered particularly from strange heart rhythms, which was a very unpleasant experience. I have had disrupted heart rhythm for a very long time, so-called arrhythmia, which I have luckily been able to keep in check through medication. During the perimenopause it worsened acutely, and I had to increase my dose of medication.

Hot flushes are not something that's made up. Far from it. It can be a very unpleasant experience and I even believe it can be confused with a panic attack or a blood pressure fall if it occurs during the day. In my case, I have been lucky enough to experience hot flushes mainly at night. But some women can feel dizzy, as if they have had a sudden drop in their blood pressure.

Hot flushes mostly occur in the night

Hot flushes can last for anything from a few seconds to a couple of minutes, may appear once during the night or fifty times during the day. So, as I said, it's very individual, but researchers have still been able to find a few commonalities. For example, hot flushes often appear between one o'clock and three o'clock at night. Many women lie awake exactly at these hours, which could be because of the hot flushes. It's also hard to say at which age hot flushes appear. But what seems to be common is that they sneak up on you at the start of the perimenopause, and then occur more often as you get closer to the menopause.

There may also be a connection between more hot flushes and being overweight, smoking, alcohol, sleeplessness, caffeine, stress, and too much carbohydrates. Scientists, however, are not completely agreed on the causes, and it's hard to tell if you have more hot flushes due to being overweight or if it depends upon other factors in your lifestyle. Several studies have, on the other hand, shown that smoking can affect your symptoms during the perimenopause, so giving up smoking is a good first step. I even have friends who have given up coffee and alcohol and feel that their hot flushes have reduced or even stopped altogether.

Hot flushes and sleeplessness are closely linked, but it's not always the hot flushes that cause the sleeplessness. It is, however, safe to say that the aftermath (sweating) of a hot flush *always* wakes you up. In other words, one thing leads to another. At the same time, some of us don't get hot flushes, instead we just can't sleep and are feeling low.

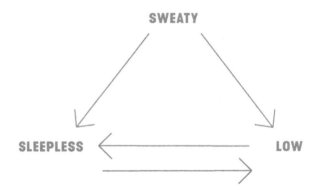

Sleep is essential for body and mind

What I found the worst to endure was the inability to sleep, and for me this was partly caused by hot flushes. It's no myth that a lack of sleep can drive you mad, even if media sometimes tries to make out that people can work with no or very little sleep. There is even a term for this that I have read in many international health publications: the sleepless elite – as if not sleeping were a merit.

Merit not to sleep? – No!

But it's not good not to sleep. Having a good sleep pattern is essential. Not just because a lack of sleep can lead to poor mental health, but also because it's dangerous from a physiological perspective. Sleep is needed for the body and the brain to recover and process experiences. The need for sleep differs between different people, but you could say that a grown adult generally needs between six and nine hours of sleep to be well-rested.

Scientists from, for example, Oxford, Cambridge, and Harvard, have all concluded that, on average, we sleep two hours less today than we did in the 1960s and that, as a consequence, our health has suffered. One scientist even claimed that a lack of sleep is as bad as sugar and can be seen as the next big health hazard of our time.

During sleep, a growth hormone is released helping insulin to store sugar. If this is disrupted, the storage of the sugar doesn't work that well. After just a couple of days, too much sugar will be circulating in your blood and after a week you will have levels that can be comparable to a diabetic. Diabetes is an illness that can also affect your heart in the end. So, if you raise the risk of diabetes, the risk of heart and vascular disease also goes up.

When you stop sleeping, you are also at risk of depression and burnout. Both depression and burnout are reactions to long-term stress, and lack of sleep is enormously stressful for your body.

How long can you cope without sleeping? A rat can cope without sleep for 4–5 weeks before it dies. Far less time is needed for you to become a zombie. Nobody really knows how long a human being can go without sleeping before they die, but the holder of the Guinness World Record of being awake the longest time is a 17-year-old student who did not sleep for 264 hours. For 11 days he was completely awake. After that he slept for just over 14 hours and appeared completely restored. This is, however, not something I recommend you try.

There are, above all, two hormones that affect sleep. One is cortisol, which is a stress and alertness hormone, which makes us feel awake and full of energy, and the other is melatonin – our sleep hormone.

We are all programmed with a daily rhythm, also known as a circadian rhythm. It's about 24 hours long, that is, as long as a day. The circadian rhythm affects the production of both cortisol and melatonin.

The daily rhythm is regulated by an interaction in your brain, and the body's manufacturing of melatonin is stimulated by darkness. This makes you sleep better when it's dark, and normally you don't have a problem staying awake when it's

TWO HORMONES THAT AFFECT YOUR SLEEP

Cortisol: a hormone that makes you alert and gives you energy.

Melatonin: a hormone that makes you sleepy.

light outside. For a healthy person, the cortisol peaks in the morning and before lunch, when you need energy the most to get going. Then the cortisol decreases throughout the day to be at its lowest level in the evening and at night.

Melatonin is a sleep hormone that makes you feel tired and helps you to go to sleep and remain asleep throughout the night. The level of melatonin is at its highest during the evening and at night. When you enter the perimenopause and the hormones start to change, your stress and sleep hormones are affected too.

Some people suffer from reduced cortisol levels and find it difficult to get up in the morning. Some people dip at two or three o'clock in the afternoon. Others have too little melatonin when going to sleep.

The levels of cortisol and melatonin also change during the perimenopause, and with age and possibly raised stress levels, the melatonin decreases in both men and women. Too little melatonin causes us not going into a deep sleep, which makes us never feel truly well-rested. Moreover, sleep deprivation can cause many other symptoms, so let me tell you this: Sleep is the first thing you need to fix – then all other problems will be easier to handle.

Break out of the vicious circle

I hope now you have a slightly better understanding of why you may be sleepless and sweaty. But let's get to perhaps the most important part – why do you feel down? This affects us most of all. To walk around every day and not feel calm, harmonious, and happy, but instead down, sad, and low is really hard. You may be irritated and angry. You may cry and have panic attacks. Or you wake in the middle of the night feeling paranoid. You have strange thoughts about things that could happen, someone dying or becoming ill. Or that someone at work is trying to steal your position. Thoughts that simply have no bearing on reality whatsoever.

I will never forget the first time I woke up with palpitations. It was very unpleasant, and at night everything always feels extra difficult. I lay in the darkness thinking that if I fall asleep I may never wake up again. What if I am having a heart attack right now?

The thoughts that pop up in the early hours of the morning can sometimes be worrying, and it's nothing strange or unusual. But it's good to be aware that the hormone changes during the perimenopause also affect the feel-good hormones and it can become a vicious circle, for when the feel-good hormone serotonin decreases, our sleep is affected.

Worried thoughts...

In other words, swinging hormones leads to changes in serotonin levels which can lead to poor sleep. Not that strange, then, that we feel low and have problems sleeping. A lack of serotonin can also bring on depression. All of these hormones seem to affect one another and therefore the entire system is disrupted.

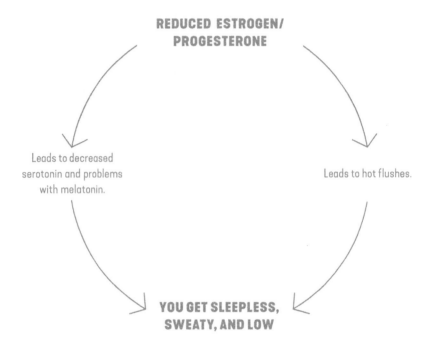

REDUCED ESTROGEN/
PROGESTERONE

Leads to decreased
serotonin and problems
with melatonin.

Leads to hot flushes.

YOU GET SLEEPLESS,
SWEATY, AND LOW

As you can see, sleep is central to your well-being. It's important that you get it sorted out. It's also important to get help if you can't sleep since you could be suffering from something that requires medication. In some cases, it may be enough to fix your swinging hormones, which is the main purpose of this book. Don't worry. Soon you will get all the inspiration you need to do what suits you best when the symptoms bother you the most. There is always something you can do and don't forget: your perimenopower is with you.

CHAPTER 6

Don't worry

If you feel the same as I that you will eventually do ANYTHING not to have these strange symptoms, you have come to the right place. For I have some good news. The first, and possibly most important, thing you can do to relieve the hormonal unease in your body is to take care of it from the inside out. I am sure you've read masses about miracle diets and training programs to get into top physical shape, perhaps with the main purpose of fitting into the norm of how you »should« look. But the fact is that training and the right diet, more than anything else, will make you FEEL BETTER, even during the perimenopause. It's not exactly rocket science, but it's good to be reminded about it every now and then to give yourself the chance to focus on *why* you need to look after your body.

Dare to try something new

For a long time, I found it hard to pull myself together when I was feeling awful. I was both worried and frustrated about all the strange things that were happening, and the last thing I wanted to do was to go out jogging. It would feel so much better to sit on the couch with my hand reaching into a packet of crisps instead. Do you recognize this in yourself?

But maybe it's time to try something new. Regardless of how well you look after your body in your current situation, you might feel better if you change something in your lifestyle. After all, everything in life is connected, and even though your mental well-being is largely influenced by external factors like the weather, your finances, and your relationships with your boss, partner, or parents, it's amazing how much we can affect our bodies with the help of what we put in our mouths and how much we exercise.

All our symptoms are also connected. If you have night sweats, it affects your sleep. If you sleep badly, you feel low. If you are low, it can be hard to look after yourself properly. But breaking the downward spiral is easier than you think, if you know what to do.

Small changes make a big difference

In Part Two – The Help is Here – you will learn what I did to lessen my troubles, and all other chapters follow the same theme. Yes, your guess is right: food and exercise. During the first years of my perimenopause, I realized that this was my savior, it was the »medicine« that had the greatest influence on how I felt. After all, the body is a machine and if we look after it correctly with regular sleep, healthy food, and physical activity, it will continue to work optimally, even during the perimenopause.

Now don't misunderstand me, I don't mean that you necessarily have to make a complete change and become a fitness fanatic living solely on vegetable smoothies. (If you do choose to go all-in with that lifestyle, go for it!) But what I want to say is that, regardless of where in life you are right now, you may witness miracles just by taking an extra walk every now and then. A power walk is a great recipe for kick-starting your perimenopower!

>>Training is a
good drug. Become
addicted to it and
you'll feel better,
you'll see ...<<

A TEXT MESSAGE FROM ONE OF MY DOCTOR FRIENDS

By changing your lifestyle, you can provide your body with the best conditions for regaining its balance. But if that's not enough for you, I have a few aces up my sleeve, or at least, further on in the book. You see, I want you to know *everything*, absolutely everything you need to know to find out how you can get help. I don't want you to worry, sooner or later you will try something that will work wonders for you and you won't have to wake up sweaty and confused at night.

If you look upon this period as a time in your life when you will think more about yourself than before, then you are on the right road to finding your perimenopower. More care and more love towards yourself are the first things you need during the initial years when the hormones begin to change. If you give yourself the best conditions, I believe it will be easier for you. I believe you are just like me. You just want the hardship to go away. If so, I want to congratulate you for you have come to the right place. In the following chapter, I will show you which keys I used to unlock my perimenopower. I knew it was there, I just hadn't seen it for a very long time.

Give yourself some love!

Part 2

The Help is Here

»I slept two
hours last night
and three the night
before, but it doesn't
matter as long as I
can catch up in the
weekend.«

TEXT MESSAGE FROM ONE OF MY FRIENDS

CHAPTER 7

Sleep like a queen

The root of much of the evil in the perimenopause is disturbed sleep. I would like to say it's the root of all evil. Sleeplessness isn't something you can ignore, it affects *your entire existence.*

When I had my first bout of sleeplessness and started talking about what I had experienced, it became apparent that many of my friends had struggled with similar problems. A friend of mine told me that she always woke up at around two or three o'clock in the night and couldn't go back to sleep, so she simply got up and baked instead. She never slept for more than five hours, not even at weekends. She is one of those people who claim not to need a lot of sleep but are able to function anyway. My answer to that is usually that it's a myth that you can cope without sleeping »that much«.

Another friend of mine told me that she felt as though she never fell into a deep sleep since she woke up every time her husband rolled over. She slept so lightly that she never felt rested. Several of my friends also told me about how they sweated so much during the night that they had to get up and take a shower. And then there is the poor friend who didn't sleep for two weeks and was admitted to a psychiatric unit – who needs to take a small white pill every day to be able to sleep so that she can function at all. She will probably have to do this for many years to come.

The human being is supposed to sleep at night. In fact, that's how we work. In the same way that you must charge your cell phone regularly, you too need to be »charged« with new energy. And five hours isn't enough, end of story. If you scrutinize yourself, how do you sleep? Do you often wake up at night, and does it take some time before you can go back to sleep? Are you sweating more than normal but haven't considered getting help for it?

Charge your body too

One way to minimize the risk of waking up sweating in the middle of the night is to have a nice, cool bedroom and a duvet that's not too warm. If that doesn't work, use my tips below and if none of those help, you should, of course, seek medical advice.

Everything starts with a good night's sleep

Perhaps, like me, you are thinking that on a normal night you fall asleep just like that – bam! – and then wake up – bam! – completely rested and amazing. But now I have learned that it's a little more complicated than that.

Over the course of a normal night, we sleep in several consecutive *sleep cycles*. Each cycle lasts for around an hour and a half, and throughout the cycle we sleep both deeply and lightly. When the sleep cycle is finished, we wake up for a few seconds before the next one starts, but we hardly ever remember this. It may sound strange, since we don't remember the micro-awakening, but it's true. I have even heard that you need to be awake for up to five minutes to be able to remember it afterwards.

But despite sleeping more lightly in periods throughout

the night, we are not made to wake up over and over just because our partner snores or rolls over next to you. We shouldn't have to change sheets in the middle of the night either. If you constantly wake up, you never enter the deep sleep the body needs to recover properly. Luckily, there is help to be found. I have tried everything, and I would like to share what I have found useful. Hopefully something will work for you too.

1 AVOID CAFFEINE

I have had the best effect on my sleep when I have stopped drinking coffee altogether. Caffeine has a stimulating effect and therefore a complete break from caffeine can make a huge difference in the way you feel and, above all, how you sleep. But if you, like many others, find it hard to function normally without your morning coffee, consider letting the first cup of the day also be your last. Try it for a week and see if you experience any difference in how well you sleep.

2 EXERCISE

Exercise increases your feel-good endorphins and can help you sleep better. When I am in a period where I exercise regularly, it becomes very obvious that I sleep better than during periods when I exercise less. My brain is no longer in overdrive, because I feel that when the body is tired, my brain doesn't have the energy to cause me any trouble.

On the other hand, during the periods when I haven't exercised, I have felt as though my thoughts are like an old scratched record. I lie in bed thinking so much that I can't relax and then I can't sleep at all.

I have also noticed that exercising too close to bedtime is not to be recommended. When you exercise, your body gets energized before it can start to relax, so you will need sufficient time to unwind. I try to avoid exercising after eight o'clock at night, which works well for me.

When you have tried exercising, cut out the coffee, and sleep in a cool room, but still have trouble sleeping, what is the next step?

 ## YOGA

Start a beginner's course or look for yoga instructions online. Do a couple of yoga exercises at home every day for a month – fifteen minutes at a time is enough. I promise that you will start sleeping better. But perhaps you have already tried yoga and feel that it's not your cup of tea. Maybe you are like my friend, who glared at me and said:

– Katarina, if you tell me one more time to start yoga so I can sleep again, I´m going to break up with you.

We laughed and realized that she was probably not in the yoga phase. I completely understand that – not everyone wants to do yoga and many people feel it's far too slow. But the fact is, yoga makes the body relax, and in my case, it felt as though yoga pulled me out of the state of tension I felt I was in.

There is a particular type of yoga which I found incredibly useful for improving my sleep. I even used to call it sleep yoga. Every Friday at three o'clock, I went to a class

»Katarina,
if you tell me
one more time to
start yoga so I can
sleep again, I'm
going to break up
with you.«

CONVERSATION WITH ONE OF MY BEST FRIENDS

called Restorative Yoga. The idea was that you would lie in relaxing positions for a very long time with the help of bolsters, cushions, and warm blankets. It wasn't about getting sweaty or doing handstands. It was about relaxation, the deepest kind of relaxation you could ever imagine. I can't even describe what went on during those 90 minutes. During some classes, it felt like I was somewhere between being asleep and awake.

Yoga for a good night's sleep

After a class like that, I was so incredibly relaxed, but at the same time I felt like I had an extreme regeneration of energy. I was exhausted yet at the same time so alert. During my terrible insomnia period, I knew that I would sleep better in the weekend if I went to my sleep yoga. After those classes I had at least two sleep-filled nights in a row.

Yoga helped me and I hope that you, even if you are not there yet, some day will get to the yoga phase. And I hope you will get the chance to try something like sleep yoga.

But if exercise, yoga, and giving up caffeine doesn't help, there are other things to try. For when I have decided to do something, or to help someone, I don't normally give up. My view is that there is always another way.

4 ACUPRESSURE MAT

The acupressure mat is a relaxing product originating from yoga. An acupressure mat is a mat, with hundreds of tiny spikes, whose only function is that you should lie on it. I understand if you think it sounds strange, I did too. But acupressure mats have been used by people who practice yoga since the dawn of time, and when one of my close friends started to rave about the acupressure mat, I decided to try it.

Just as you might think when lying down on a bed of tiny nails, it hurts. But it also gets your blood circulation going and, in a strange way, it calms your body down. The mat has a relaxing effect particularly during times of stress.

During one period, I would lie down on my mat in bed at night and fall asleep on it. Although it hurt, it was as if the pain made the body focus on relaxing. In the end, I fell asleep. During my worst periods of sleeplessness, I even brought my mat with me in my suitcase, so I could sleep better when I was away.

The acupressure mat is said to generate a state of deep relaxation and the fact is, it worked for me. Sure, I woke up to remove the mat, but I often went straight back to sleep. And if I woke in the middle of the night I would sometimes get it out again.

 EVENING BATH

Another thing that I made a habit of when I couldn't sleep was to run a bath. I lit scented candles, added some lavender oil and floated in darkness for half an hour. To combine warmth and water, just like in a uterus, pleasantly relaxes your body, and lavender oil has a beneficial effect in calming your senses. On many occasions, I have fallen fast asleep after such a treatment.

If you like going to the spa, you will know exactly what I mean. Sometimes a calm and warm environment is all your body needs to let go of the tension, so you can relax and fall asleep.

I hope you will sleep better after trying my tips. Wouldn't it be wonderful to discover that, as long as you are kind to your body, allowing it to unwind, you will become friends? For this is what it feels like when you are right in the middle of your worst phase. Like you have fallen out with your own body and you are prepared to do anything to become friends again.

During the first years of the perimenopause, when the hormones first began to fight each other, the things I've mentioned above were enough for me to become calmer. But the closer I got to menopause, the more apparent my troubles became, and I attempted to enter the world of supplements and unprescribed medication.

I would like to advise you about the ones that I found most useful to me, but I want to make it clear that I am not a doctor and that the medication that worked for me may not work as well for you and your body. Nothing beats the personal advice and care provided by your medical center or gynecologist. Therefore, my aim isn't to recommend these supplements, it's just to introduce you to a few of those that are available so that you will *know there is help* and that sometimes that help is packaged in small jars or plastic strips. There is nothing wrong in this and many of the medicines we use are meant, as closely as possible, to mimic the vitamins, hormones, or other substances we have naturally in our bodies but which, for some reason, we need another dose of.

I also want to make the point that I am not an advocate of stuffing my body full of medicine, as I am sure you have already understood. I am completely convinced that the biggest changes come from our lifestyle, the sort of things I mentioned in bullets 1–5. Bullets 6–8 on my sleep guide are aimed at those who have more severe problems where none of the above provide a good enough effect.

NATURAL SUPPLEMENTS

In health food stores, there are natural supplements that have a calming effect and may help you to start sleeping again. One example is *valerian*. It's a perennial herb that grows in both Europe and Asia. Another natural remedy with a calming effect is a trendy newcomer in the health food business, the herb *ashwagandha*. Both valerian and ashwagandha are calming and used to treat anxiety. Many people take valerian in order to sleep or to relax, and if your sleep problems are moderate, valerian can help. I used valerian during the day for a while and didn't feel as wound-up. Ashwagandha is said to have the same effect, but I haven't tried it for a long enough period myself to notice any significant difference to my sleep.

MELATONIN

Another medicine, or rather hormone, that I would like to mention is melatonin. Melatonin is the hormone that's the most important to our sleep. It's produced naturally in the body and makes our bodies understand when it's day and when it's night. With age, the production of melatonin decreases, and it can also decrease during periods of severe stress. If you have other hormone problems, the level decreases even further. If the level decreases, you will have trouble sleeping, and moreover, melatonin has also shown to be important to our feel-good hormones. Just like the sex hormone estrogen.

Just let me sleep!

So, if both melatonin and estrogen decrease, there can be no other result than you having trouble sleeping. And if that also affects our feel-good hormone, serotonin, the result is that we sleep badly *and* we feel down. Of course, it's difficult to know if you are feeling low because you are sleeping badly, or if you are sleeping badly because you are feeling low. So, it's not just a restless mind and hot flushes that cause sleep problems, it can also be due to your level of sleep hormones having been disrupted.

In August 2017, a major British meta-analysis was conducted where a research team compared 5,030 studies to determine if conclusions could be drawn on the real effects of melatonin. In other words, if melatonin as a supplement was effective against sleeplessness. It showed that melatonin has a clear effect on those who can't sleep compared to placebo patients (patients who *thought* they had taken the medicine but had actually just taken a sugar pill).

In Europe and the US, melatonin is sold like any other vitamin, while in Sweden it's still under much debate. It's argued that, just because it's natural, doesn't mean it's good. This, of course, is true – not everything natural is necessarily good.

But it's interesting that the view on melatonin differs so much throughout the world, and that some countries are more restrictive than others.

I have spoken to Professor Torbjörn Åkerstedt who had many interesting things to say about sleeping and melatonin. When I asked him why he doesn't think melatonin is that popular as a medicine in some parts of the world, he answered that the reason might be that melatonin is natural and therefore it can't be patented. In other words, there is no money for research or profit, so few people will want to invest money in producing it.

Torbjörn also mentioned research that shows that melatonin is not just good for your sleep but is also proven to have anti-cancer effects that counteract mutations in the cells. But, on the other hand, there are studies that show that melatonin is more or less without side effects, good or bad.

Melatonin decreases with age, and if exercise, sleep yoga, and natural remedies don't help you sleep better, melatonin may be an option. If it proves to give you other health benefits as well, that's just a bonus. It's not without reason that melatonin is known as a miracle drug in the US.

8 ATARAX

Once I started to sleep better but still felt anxious now and again, I asked my gynecologist if she could suggest something that helped with anxiety and made my body relax. For even if I could sleep, my body sometimes felt tense as though I was unable to wind down. Have you ever felt like that?

I made it clear that I wanted to avoid anti-depressants, sleeping pills, and anxiety suppressants. I asked for an alternative that you could not become addicted to but could just take now and then. She suggested I try Atarax. Even though, overall, I am very dubious about using medication if it can be avoided, I would like to tell you about how Atarax worked for me and why I tried it at all.

Atarax is a medicine given, for example, to small children to ease the itching of chicken pox. It blocks histamine, a substance that can sometimes cause allergic reactions in certain cells. Atarax has also shown to work against anxiety and worry since it makes your muscles relax but has no proven effect on sleeping problems. It's also not addictive.

To me, Atarax is so relaxing that I fall asleep. I take the smallest dose, 10mg, and for me that's enough. I have taken it when I have felt uneasy and worried and sometimes if I have slept badly for a two nights in a row. On the third night, I can take an Atarax to finally get a good night's sleep. When things were at their worst for me, having melatonin and Atarax was a great comfort.

Do the easiest things first

Now I have given you eight tips on how to improve your sleep. I believe and hope that this will work well for you. If you are just like I was, willing to try anything, hopefully these tips will help you on your way. At least I hope they will help you to get a good night's sleep every now and then. For now, maybe you only need these tips for a couple of days per month? Maybe you sleep well except during ovulations and during your period? Maybe the menopause is still a long way ahead of you? As it comes closer, sleep problems may appear anytime and not just during ovulation and periods. And then it's important to look after yourself in every way that you can.

I have made a list with all of the above tips. I recommend you try them in order. If your sleeping problems are severe, you may not find a solution until you are way down the list. If your sleep problems are infrequent, you might manage by using the first few tips. Anyway – off you go and sleep well!

KATARINA'S SLEEPING GUIDE

1. Avoid caffeine
2. Exercise
3. Yoga
4. Acupressure mat
5. Evening bath
6. Natural supplements
7. Melatonin
8. Atarax

CHAPTER 8

Get in the mood with food

»Let food be thy medicine and medicine be thy food.«
Hippokrates

As far back as thousands of years ago, Hippocrates coined the classic phrase, which is pertinent more now than ever. The trends of recent years are clear – food can change how you feel. Masses of scientific studies on diet are being conducted, countless books are being written, and the number of health coaches and bloggers focusing on healthy food grows every year.

I recently read about a Japanese professor who was 105 years old. His view was that you should »worry less about eating healthy.« This is interesting because the worry about eating healthily enough is, in itself, unhealthy. This can lead to expectations that are hard to live up to. But I still feel that if you are ever going to try to eat more healthily, it's during this period of your life when you should be trying to take extra care of yourself. As I have said before, this is a phase when many things are happening within your body and if you are aware of it and give your body the right type of »fuel« it will work the way you want it to. This chapter will be about how food affects your perimenopausal symptoms.

Sometimes when I eat spicy food I begin to sweat, the heat in the mouth seems to affect the rest of the body too. Does this sound familiar?

Food has a greater effect than you think

Sometimes I feel there are so many new findings that I can hardly keep track of them. It's not always easy knowing what is best for you, and some say that food plays an extremely important role while others say it doesn't matter as much as you think. But there are several examples that indicate that food plays an important role in perimenopausal symptoms.

Asian women, for example, report far less problems with hot flushes than Western women. The theories on why it's like that vary, but many believe the reason to be the Asians' enormous consumption of soy. Soy contains *phytoestrogen* – a plant material similar to the estrogen produced naturally in the body. Since Asian women eat a lot of soy, there are theories that the phytoestrogens in soy have an effect on the likelihood of suffering hot flushes. But the phytoestrogen is so weak in soy that it would take a complete change in diet for us Westerners to be able to benefit from it. In other words, a whole lot of tofu. But it's still interesting that diet affects the symptoms so clearly.

Cultural differences

Another food category that affects health is spicy food. Sometimes when I eat spicy food I begin to sweat, the heat in the mouth seems to affect the rest of the body too. Does this sound familiar? Since one of our most common symptoms during the perimenopause is sweating, it might be a good idea to avoid hot, spicy food during your perimenopause if this is a particular problem for you.

It's also interesting to see a connection between health and meat consumption. There have been several studies over the past few years showing that a plant-based diet is healthier than a meat-based one. The World Health Organization (WHO) has even distributed a warning that processed meat products can be as dangerous to your health as smoking. It may seem strange that something most of us eat every day can be so harmful. But there may be something to it.

Eat less meat

An American study with over 90,000 respondents showed that vegetarian diets led to a decreased risk of heart and vascular diseases, high blood pressure, type 2 diabetes, and some forms of cancer. A British study with over 65,000 respondents had the same result. Conversely, the risks increased when regularly eating large amounts of meat. Yet it's still very difficult for many of us to switch the beef casserole to a vegetarian equivalent.

I never used to pay much attention to what I ate on a day-to-day basis. I was often under a lot of stress and worked long hours and constantly felt guilty about the children. I always made sure they got lots of good, nutritious food, but I neglected myself. Frequently, I didn't have time for breakfast and instead ate something quickly in front of my computer. There were many quick carbohydrates and I could go for long periods without thinking about what I put in my mouth. But somewhere in the back of my head, I started to wonder how my future health was going to be affected by what I did to my body.

I love food and see it as one of the big pleasures in life. I love going to good restaurants and one of my favorite meals is steak tartar. But I don't eat steak tartar every day. When it comes to food I believe in the word »moderation.« I fully respect all types of diet and food preferences, but I believe that a balanced diet in »moderation« may be just what the body needs. So, here is a chapter about what kinds of food helped me to feel better during my perimenopause.

Vegetarian food can minimize the symptoms

When I heard about the positive effects vegetarian food has on your health, I decided to eat solely vegetarian food for a couple of months. I wanted to find out if the claims about meat were right.

I measured my cholesterol levels before I started, ate vegetarian food for three months (I'll be honest and confess to cheating a few times with salmon), and measured my cholesterol levels again. Although my levels were good before the diet change, they were even better after I stopped eating meat. I also noticed that my perimenopausal symptoms had decreased. I rarely suffered night sweats and, when I did, it was normally during my period. Nowadays I eat a little meat again. Still, I rarely cook meat at home, but if I am invited out and beef casserole is served, I will eat it.

I strive to live a healthy lifestyle and try to avoid junk food with a lot of fat and sugar, and I noticed that, with my small changes, my symptoms decreased. Before, it felt as though I had a problem with my blood sugar. It went up and down along with my mood. Now I don't feel these variations anymore. Blood sugar levels are more stable when you don't eat food rich in sugar or carbohydrates. Many women have blood sugar problems during this period without having diabetes, and I was one of them. If I didn't eat every three hours I felt shaky. I also felt extremely tired after each meal as if eating took away energy from me in a way that I hadn't felt before.

The mood swings!

All of this is connected to sex hormone changes. When there is a dispute in the sex hormone camp, other hormones are also affected. There is research being conducted today on what happens to your body during these times, but what is known is that changes in estrogen seems to indirectly affect blood sugar.

Letting go of sugar has been hard for me but I have had to do it. I was not feeling good because of my large sugar intake, which came from eating sugar several times per week, mainly in the form of sweets, chocolate, and ice cream. But when I cut down on white sugar, I felt a significant difference. I haven't been picky about the »hidden« sugar, for example in ketchup, muesli, bread, and such things, but I have tried cutting out sweets at least during the week.

Of course, it's important to have carbohydrates, but try to choose the so-called slow carbohydrates that take longer for the body to absorb into the blood, which doesn't create the quick »sugar rush« that comes from carbohydrates found in ice cream, sweets, bread, and pasta. Slow carbohydrates, however, give a longer feeling of fullness and are found in, among other things, beans, brown pasta, and brown rice.

Don't give up!

In the middle of the period when I was feeling at my worst and having problems sleeping, I found it very hard to think about eating healthily. My body was in overdrive and I sometimes felt that I could hardly keep my head above water. All I wanted was to eat junk food, skip exercise, and just go to bed.

When you are not sleeping, your body is under extreme stress; you are tired, yet your body is in overdrive. The less you sleep, the higher the level of stress, which in turn leads to a larger appetite. Did you know that many people eat junk food when they are stressed out? This is partly because they lack the energy to cook healthy food, partly because the body is crying out for quick energy, which you get from junk food. No wonder my body was crying out for fast carbohydrates which would give me energy when I hadn't slept.

I also noticed that, when I slept and ate badly, I slowly but surely started gaining weight. Even when I exercised and ate as I have always done, I gained weight. I thought that this was odd until I learnt that, during the perimenopause, your metabolism slows down, making it easier to gain weight. So, don't worry if you suddenly start gaining weight without having made any major changes to your lifestyle – it's completely normal. But, it's yet another reason to think about whether you need to change something in your daily routine to make up for your decreased metabolism. Maybe you can manage on smaller portions than before, since you are using less energy?

All I wanted was
to eat junk food,
skip exercise,
and just go to bed.

A consequence of weight gain can be an increase in peri-menopausal problems. Some studies have shown that those with high cholesterol (which is often connected with being overweight) often suffer more from hot flushes and sweating than others. If you, like me, start eating more plant-based food, your cholesterol levels can improve, and you may experience fewer problems. If you care about what goes on in your body and put your mind to it, you will at least minimize the risk of problems. Once I understood the connection between food, sleep, and weight, it inspired me to be kind to my body in order to set things right.

Easier to gain weight

I also noticed other symptoms directly connected to my diet. For example, I experienced palpitations when I drank too much coffee or alcohol, which I had never experienced before. My body told me clearly that something wasn't right. I hadn't listened to my body before but now it was time to do so. I concluded that if I exercised more and ate better I would find my superpower again. So, I tried to do everything within my power to find my way among the different diets and theories.

My interpretation of the numerous studies, articles, books, and blogs I have read, together with the results of my own experience, is that the diet with the best effect on perime-nopausal symptoms is the so-called Mediterranean diet. It's a balanced diet that isn't so much about what you cut out, but rather about eating a little of everything and, above all, things that provide long-term energy rather than quick energy. You even eat red meat with the Mediterranean diet, but far less of it. It's reminiscent of the Nordic diet: a lot of fruit and vegetables, nuts and almonds, pulses, vegetable oils, whole grains and fish, and less red meat, milk, and dairy produce.

Hamburgers, chips (french fries), sausages, sweets, and ice-cream are a few examples of what we call junk food. How do you feel when you have had salmon and salad compared to when you have eaten a burger with bread and dressing? If you cut out the junk food your fat storage within your body decreases and if you add healthy greens and a lot of protein, you will feel much better.

Do you need supplements?

Minor changes here and there can do a lot of all-round good. My advice is for your diet to contain mainly: protein, fiber, fruit and vegetables, and healthy fats such as nuts, avocado, and olive oil. Be careful with carbohydrates and dairy produce. Nowadays most of these can be replaced with, for example, soy and oat products. Avoid sugar and cut down on meat (especially red meat) and junk food such as processed foods and fast food. If you don't get enough vitamins from your food, you may need to think about supplements.

Some doctors say that you don't need to take supplements unless you have any deficiencies, in other words illnesses brought about by abnormally low levels of vitamins or other essentials that your body really needs. However, vegans are recommended to take an extra supplement of iron and vitamin B12 as these can be difficult to get from a completely vegan diet. There are also those who recommend a supplement of omega 3 if you, for example, don't eat fish.

Personally, I have used supplements over certain periods. For example, there was a time when I often had infections in my body which led me to take extra vitamin c. In Sweden, for example, we have many dark months and therefore it may be a good idea to take additional vitamin D to compensate for the lack of sun.

During the perimenopause, I have also chosen to help my body by taking a few more supplements. My gynecologist recommended that I take vitamin B, especially B6. Vitamin B6 is needed for the brain cells to function normally, and a lack of vitamin B can cause you to feel low and irritated. A lack of vitamin B12 can even increase the risk of depression. Therefore, adding vitamin B can make you feel less down during perimenopause.

I also take magnesium supplements, which is a mineral. A lack of magnesium can, as well as some physical symptoms, also cause psychological problems such as depression or mental tiredness. Several dietitians claim that you sleep better if you take magnesium and, since this has been my biggest problem, I choose to take it.

My own experiences tell me that Hippocrates may have been right. What if food can be our medicine? And that if we start to think about what we eat, we can minimize the risk of perimenopausal problems?

B6

is found mainly in animal-based food, but also in potatoes, grains, and berries. Among other things, the vitamin is very important for the function of the nerves.

B12

is plentiful in animal-based products. Fish, meat, and shellfish, for example, contain high levels of B12. Vegans are recommended to take a supplement of B12 as it's an important vitamin that you should not be deficient in. The vitamin is needed for metabolism within the cells and the production of blood cells but is also said to have an important function for the nervous system.

VITAMIN C

is our best-known vitamin, the one that everyone talks about. It's an antioxidant that, among other things, helps to keep us healthy. It's found in most vegetables, berries, and fruits.

VITAMIN D

is needed for strong bones, teeth, and immune system. It also affects our mood. We get it in two ways: from the sun and from certain foods such as fish, dairy products, and eggs.

IRON

Among other things, iron is needed to transport oxygen from your lungs to your tissues. There is a lot of iron in meat and offal. There is also plenty of iron in pulses and bananas, and green vegetables such as spinach and broccoli. If you are unsure about whether you consume enough iron, a simple blood test at your medical center will measure your iron levels.

MAGNESIUM

is found in pulses, leafy vegetables, whole grains, meat, and fish and is needed for normal nerve and muscles function.

»After a spinning session I feel at my best. It feels like all my problems are suddenly blown away.«

PERNILLA, 43

CHAPTER 9

Training makes you tougher

I started to suspect a connection between exercise and the perimenopause when a close friend of mine, who was about to turn 40, suddenly couldn't maintain her weight. She had always exercised and eaten healthily but, without having made any changes, she started to put on weight. Her mental state grew worse and she felt very low. On top of this, she also started having problems with her sleep. What was she doing wrong?

Interestingly, our conclusion was that she was exercising far too often and too hard. Too intensively. For when she started combining her exercising with slower sessions and tweaked her diet, she started to lose weight, sleep better, and felt much more energized. My conclusion was that the problems she had been experiencing were connected to her hormones having started to change. Intense training, that she had earlier managed without any difficulty, now caused her problems. In her case, the solution was to train less often and less intensively.

I am the sort of person who needs to put in maximum

effort to find exercising fun. In other words, I love high-intensity interval sessions or long spinning sessions that exhaust me completely. I have never even considered that this might be bad for my body. But after my friend began feeling better when cutting down on her exercising, I started to think more about how training affects perimenopausal symptoms, and that it might not be as simple as the more training the better.

Exercising too intensively can raise stress levels

When exercising, the stress levels in your body temporarily increase. After exercising, the stress levels decrease again – they even go down to a lower level than before exercising. But since you are more sensitive to stress during the perimenopause, it can be more difficult than usual for your body to determine what causes this stress and which "actions" the brain should take. All of this becomes stressful and, as the stress hormones increase, the progesterone and estrogen levels decrease.

not too much, not too little

Bearing in mind that hormones naturally decrease during the perimenopause, maybe it's not such a good idea to do things that lower the levels even more. Perhaps it's sensible to cancel the marathon if you are in a difficult period. I do want to remind you that everything is individual and, if you feel good about training for a marathon, of course you should continue to do so. But if you have started to notice problems and you exercise a lot, it might be worth trying to reduce the training to see if you notice any difference.

In the American magazine *Fitness Journal*, there is a compilation of several studies on »Training Through the Transition,« in other words exercising during the perimenopause, in which many scientists agree that pulse-raising activity of a medium intensity is better than high-intensity. And the more studies I have read, the more I realize that there might be advantages to exercising more gently during the perimenopause. At least if you have problems with your sleep. Many believe that exercising makes you exert yourself, therefore tiring you out, but it's not just down to that. As previously mentioned, exercising vigorously can increase the stress levels in your body leading to it taking longer for your body to relax. If you feel more tired than usual, you should slow down. During the perimenopause when your body is overstrained, what it needs is more calm and tranquility, not more stress.

If you already exercise hard, be observant if you feel too high afterwards. If this is the case, you should combine your intensive sessions with gentler ones. If you don't have the energy to exercise, be grateful every time you do manage it.

During my perimenopause, I noticed that I slept worse having done a spinning session late at night. I could not wind down. When I did gentler exercise sessions instead, such as Pilates or light-weight training, it was far easier to get to sleep.

I want to stress that the best training session is the one that actually happens. But do remember that how much you need to exercise in order to notice a difference in your symptoms is individual, and what you do matters less – the most important

When we exercise,
endorphins are
released which makes
us feel good. It's so
powerful that, during a
period when I exercised
a lot, I felt worse
when I didn't.

thing is that you do something. Some people run marathons a couple of times per year, others are satisfied going to the gym once in a while. Just remember to listen to your body and maybe try something new now and again to see if there is any difference in how you feel.

Exercising is our best medicine

Anders Hansen, chief physician in psychiatry and author of several books, insists time and time again that exercising is like a hundred medicines. In his book *Brain Power* (2016), he explains how exercising affects our brain. One of his theses is that, in today's society, we find it hard to eliminate stress and that we instead should focus on becoming more stress resistant. And the best way to do this, according to him, is to exercise, especially any exercise that raises your pulse. There are parts of the brain that work to slow down stress, and research shows that these parts grow when we exercise.

What Hansen means is that, through exercise, we can change how our brain works, and thereby influence our mood and well-being. Isn't it great that we have the power to make such an impact? That makes me, at least, more motivated to get out on the running track.

Another thing that exercise does is increase one of your body's feel-good hormones – the endorphins. When we exercise, endorphins are released which makes us feel good. It's so powerful that, during a period when I exercised a lot, I felt worse when I didn't. Exercising had almost become an addiction.

If exercising can have such a significant effect on your brain and give such positive effects to decrease stress, it's not hard to think one step further; that training has a calming and uplifting effect on what you experience during the perimenopause. I understand that it can be hard to take in the fact that you should exercise while suffering from all sorts of difficult symptoms, when all you are trying to do is keep your head above water. But I believe that regular physical activity is one of the best things you can do to feel better at this time, and much research supports this. Since sleeping problems and mood swings are problems that we want to nip in the bud during the perimenopause, it speaks for itself that exercise is exactly what we should be doing.

It has also shown that exercising helps against hot flushes and sweating. Mats Hammar, professor emeritus in gynecology and obstetrics at Linköping University, was the first in the world to demonstrate that exercising reduced certain symptoms connected to the menopause (the time when your periods *end*), especially hot flushes and sweating.

One of his theories is that the »thermostat« in the brain that regulates body temperature doesn't work properly, therefore giving hot flushes and sweating. The thermostat is connected to the level of endorphins in your body, and the endorphin level decreases as the estrogen decreases. Because of the estrogen reduction, the thermostat believes the body is too hot and sends out blood to the extremities, which sends out heat. This activates the sweat glands in order to lower the body's temperature. In other words, everything is completely confused.

Now to the really interesting part. Since the level of endorphins directly affects the thermostat's ability to accurately regulate the body's temperature, perhaps the temperature would be more accurately regulated if the endorphin levels increased. Wouldn't it be practical if we could influence the release of endorphins somehow …? Luckily, Mats Hammar has already figured it out for us.

Mats's study showed that exercising women generally had less symptoms during the menopause, and he concluded that exercise might very well help, especially when the symptoms are to do with sweating and hot flushes. Among other things, physical activity releases a type of endorphin that contributes to the regulation of body temperature. It's a very interesting study that received much attention since it was the first of its kind.

ESTROGEN DECREASES

1 The endorphins become unsettled and endorphin levels are reduced.
2 This reduction affects the thermostat (which regulates your body temperature). The body thinks it's too hot.
3 The brain activates the sweat glands in order to lower the temperature.
4 The hot flush occurs.

There are also studies that show that after only 150 minutes per week of low-intensity exercise, many women experience fewer perimenopausal problems. You don't have to exercise more than that to realize the positive effects of exercising. For some people, three brisk 60-minute walks per week may be enough. Others want to do three weight-training sessions instead. During the perimenopause, exercising can work just like your food. It becomes your medicine. 150 minutes is less than three hours of the 168 hours in the week. If it helps you to overcome your problems and make your daily life easier, surely that can be considered time well invested.

Only 150 minutes a week!

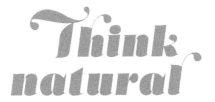

CHAPTER 10

Think natural

Now you know how to sort out your sleep, what to eat, and how to exercise to feel your best. These are the easiest things you can do to feel better. But if you still have problems after trying my suggestions, I would like you to try natural health food.

From nature or the lab – what is best?

You could say that health foods are a step between groceries and so-called traditional or Western medicine. Apart from the positive effects that the right groceries in your everyday food can give you, there is health food in the form of herbs and plants that have been used throughout time in addition to food to cure or ease different illnesses and ailments. You could look at health food as our »medicine« before there were laboratories that chemically could »concoct« a mixture of the exact ingredients needed to cure illnesses. This is why this kind of health food is sometimes called natural or alternative medicines.

One difference between health food and »normal« medicine prescribed by doctors is that the effects of the health food are not always scientifically proven. This is because there have not been as many studies on this type of medicine. But even if there isn't always scientific proof that a specific herb works on certain symptoms, many people find it effective. Could it be worth trying it yourself?

Many people believe plant-based to be better than »normal« medicines, maybe because it feels more natural to use things that grow naturally. But there are also those who are critical towards natural health foods believing it to be not as »serious« as other medicines. But in Germany, for example, the situation is different. There, alternative medicine is acknowledged as a complement to traditional medicine. In Sweden, there is still a certain skepticism toward natural remedies, even though it's more accepted today than a few years ago.

The »alternative« business turns over a great deal of money today, which suggests that we are moving towards greater acceptance. Perhaps we have been too harsh on medicinal plants that have been in use for thousands of years on other continents? Or do we need other types of medicines today than what nature can offer? Perhaps, in the past, we didn't have as much stress around us as we do today? And a completely different diet with less sugar? There were certainly no lifestyle diseases back then and perhaps it was enough to use plants to stay healthy?

I respect both sides and perhaps a combination is the best thing – take the best from both sides. And as I usually say – take in the information you need to make the right decision

»I think it's difficult
to take in which natural
remedies work, since
everybody says different
things about different
products. So, who should
I believe?«

SARA, 45

for you. But just like ordinary medicines, natural remedies can have side effects. Sometimes they can also work badly or not at all together with other medicines that you take. Like with everything, make sure that you know what you put into your body. And it's also important to bear in mind that just because it's natural, doesn't necessarily mean it's good.

Natural health food or not?

Plants in science

I have tried many natural health foods and found some that can help to ease the troubles during perimenopause. I have even had training as a health food advisor, so I have a good handle of which natural remedies are on the market. The ones I would like to present to you are the ones I have either tried or read a lot of studies about.

St John's wort

St John's wort (*Hypericum perforatum*) has been used as a remedy since medieval times and is used today to treat depression. There are studies showing that St John's wort works. For example, there was a German study in 2008 involving 5,500 patients where the result showed that St John's wort had similar effects on depression as other anti-depressant treatments, but with fewer side effects. St John's wort is, therefore, one of the herbs that can be worth trying during the perimenopause if you are feeling low.

Valerian

Valerian (*Valeriana officinalis*) is another plant that many women take during the perimenopause. Valerian is commonly taken to treat sleep problems since it has a drowsy effect. The effects of valerian are somewhat unsure but there are a couple of studies that show an effect. I have tested valerian and it calmed me down and gave me a nice feeling throughout the day.

Black cohosh

Black cohosh (*Cimicifuga racemosa*) is a plant that may have some effect on perimenopausal symptoms. The plant has been used by indigenous populations since the dawn of time to ease »women's problems.« In Germany, black cohosh has been sold as a remedy for more than 40 years, and that's where most of the research has been done. Some studies show that black cohosh has an effect while others can't find any particular connection. Those studies that show an effect say that black cohosh reduces sweating, hot flushes, irritability, depression, and sleeping problems. Absolutely everything that we want to find a cure for!

Munk's pepper

Monk's pepper (*Vitex agnus-castus*) is said to have a balancing effect on PMS and hormonal imbalance. Since the perimenopause is considered to have some symptoms in common with PMS, it may be effective to take even during this period. Many women testify that the perimenopause feels like a prolonged PMS. The difference is that PMS is over in a couple of days whereas the perimenopause remains for considerably longer than that.

In health food stores there are several products containing the plants and herbs I have mentioned above. If you are unsure of which products to try, I recommend a health food advisor who can guide you in the right direction. The business of natural remedies can be a jungle, and depending upon which health food advisor you ask, you will surely receive different answers for what will work for your symptoms. The easiest way to find out what will be best for you is to test them yourself.

There is yet another plant that appears in this context, and that's pollen extract. There are a few products containing pollen extract, but there are no major studies showing any effect on the problems, even though a few smaller studies have shown some effect.

Just as most doctors favor school medicine, health food advisors believe that you should use natural remedies. But just because it's natural, doesn't mean it's good. Be as critical towards natural remedies as you would towards school medicine. I believe a combination of natural remedies and conventional medicine might be the best. On the other hand, I don't believe you should stop a medical treatment without having discussed it first with your doctor.

I believe the most important thing is to have an open mind. There are incredible medicines that we humans have invented in laboratories, just as there are incredible herbs in nature. If you feel that you have found the right path using natural remedies, I would like to congratulate you. The rest of you can stay with me for the next chapter, for now we have arrived at the last option. Perhaps you have been holding on for several years, managing with lifestyle changes and natural remedies and feeling great, but now as you are getting towards the end of your perimenopause, suddenly you feel that it's not working one hundred percent anymore. The problems often get worse the closer you get to the menopause. But stay calm, there is still help at hand!

Keep an open mind!

»When I began
taking estrogen, I could feel
the difference after just
one day. It was as if
I had been living in a
gray fog, as if my whole
existence was muffled
until I applied that plaster.
Then it was like waking
up from a slow dream and
simply becoming normal
again.«

TESS, 45

CHAPTER 11

To take or not to take ...?

There is probably nothing within women's medicine that's more debated than estrogen. Do you have a friend with breast cancer or an older relative who tells you that estrogen is dangerous? Or did your mother take estrogen when you were a teenager? The debate about estrogen is still confusing to many. In this chapter I would like to straighten out a few question marks for you.

Estrogen – when nothing else helps

Perhaps you are in a position where you have managed to keep your perimenopause symptoms in check for several years but feel that it doesn't quite work any longer. Maybe you have tried everything I have mentioned earlier, such as exercise, changes to your diet, yoga, and natural remedies, but feel they don't help any more. You have probably reached the later phase of your perimenopause when your hormones sink to an extra low level. Further action may then be needed to reduce your problems.

When I passed the 45-year point, I noticed that certain symptoms lingered for a longer time, and I started thinking about whether it was time to begin taking an estrogen supplement. When I turned 48, I chose to begin using estrogen plasters. It's exactly what it sounds like, a plaster. It differs in size depending on the dose, and the idea is that you place it somewhere below your waist. The buttock or thigh is the perfect place. You wear it day and night which means that the estrogen is released evenly the whole time and after three to four days you change it for a new plaster.

But just like all plasters, they are attached with an adhesive that can sometimes cause irritation on your skin, especially if your skin usually is sensitive. This happened to me, so I started using estrogen gel instead. The gel is also applied to the lower part of your body, you put a thin layer on an area the size of your palm and leave it to work its way into your skin just like the plaster.

So, I chose to take estrogen when my problems became too difficult to handle in any other way. But I want to make it clear that just because I chose it, it may not be the right thing for you. It's a choice you must make based upon your own problems and whether it's worth the possible side effects.

Just like many others, I was dubious about estrogen because of the possible risks of breast cancer and heart and vascular disorders, but after going through enormous amounts of studies on the subject and becoming more know-ledgeable, I decided to give it a chance. Having read up on it properly, I concluded that the risks were probably not as big as some people wanted to set off, and I considered the advan-tages outweighing them.

Just like many others, I was dubious about estrogen because of the possible risks of breast cancer and heart and vascular disorders.

It was fascinating to see what happened when I started taking estrogen supplements. The effects were immediate. My skin changed for the better, my hair regained its volume, but above all my ability to sleep returned properly, and my mood swings disappeared (if the latter was due to my sleep being stabilized is of course a fair question). My night sweats disappeared and there was not a hint of panic attacks nor anxiety. All of a sudden, I felt completely rested, glowing, and super happy – the way I had always been deep down. My real personality came back. It really did feel as though I had been given a superpower.

New-found energy with estrogen

Many of my friends who have taken estrogen, testify to experiencing the same results. That it feels like being born again, or at least fifteen years younger. But, as with everything else: We all react differently from taking these kinds of supplements. Just as some people will feel great exercising vigorously, some will feel fantastic when taking estrogen, while others will not feel any significant difference.

Estrogen must be taken with progesterone

Once you have decided to begin taking estrogen, you must complement it with a supplement of estrogen's »hormone partner« progesterone. These two hormones make up HRT (Hormone Replacement Therapy), which is what you would commonly call treatments of estrogen and progesterone.

The reason that you must also supplement with progesterone is to prevent thickening of the endometrium. If it thickens, there is a heightened risk of cancer of the uterus. There is, however, an exception when you don't need to take proges-

HRT = HORMONE REPLACEMENT THERAPY

Hormone Replacement Therapy means short- or long-term treatment of decreasing estrogen and progesterone levels.

terone as a complement, and that is if you have removed your uterus, in which case estrogen is enough. Also, if you have had an estrogen-sensitive breast cancer, research shows that you should not take estrogen. So long as you are healthy, you can take estrogen – but as I have said earlier, it's a decision that you must make yourself.

Nowadays, estrogen supplements come in a bioidentical form, as opposed to previously when there was only a synthetic version. Because today's estrogen is bioidentical, it means that it has the same molecular structure as the body's self-produced hormone. Our body recognizes the bioidentical hormone and therefore finds it easier to deal with. You could say that the synthetic version interferes with our body, while the bioidentical one is welcomed. It rebalances the body without any greater risk of side effects.

Bioidentical estrogen is available today in the form of tablets, plasters, gel, and spray. If you take estrogen through your skin instead of in tablet form, you reduce the possible risks of side effects as the estrogen doesn't have to pass through the liver as it does when taking it as a tablet.

Attitude to estrogen – now and in the past

As little as 20 years ago it was not unusual for gynecologists to prescribe estrogen supplements. Scientists were unanimous – hormone replacement treatments protected against, among other things, heart and vascular disease. But in 2002, a study was released by the Women's Health Initiative (WHI) which changed the view on estrogen as a supplement. Instead, the study, involving 160,000 women between the ages of 50 and 79, showed that the same treatments could increase the risk of breast cancer, stroke, and heart disease.

There was also a heightened risk of ovarian cancer. The study had an enormous impact throughout the world; in Sweden the sale of estrogen is said to have more than halved. The recommendations on how to take estrogen were rewritten and the message was that the hormone treatment was only to be prescribed for short periods for acute menopausal problems.

In this study, there were several articles emphasizing the risk of breast cancer. The message was broadcast so loudly that, even in 2018, modern women still associate estrogen with breast cancer. This isn't that strange, bearing in mind that we humans are constructed to remember risks. It doesn't always matter how *big* the risks are, they are still what we focus on.

But times have changed. Lately, there has been growing criticism towards WHI's study. Of the thousands of women questioned, the average age was 63 and a third of the women were being treated for high blood pressure. So, the preconditions were not good from the start. Many of them were also overweight. In other words, there were several risk factors for becoming ill.

So, the results of the WHI study are not completely applicable for healthy women who start taking estrogen in their forties. There is also another study worth mentioning, and that is an 18-year follow-up of the women in the WHI study. The follow-up showed that the risk of death from, for example, heart and vascular disease was just as great (or small) in the group taking estrogen as the one that took the placebo.

To me, everything became clearer when I phoned the renowned professor at Uppsala University, Tord Naessén, who is regarded as the most knowledgeable person on estrogen in Sweden. After our conversation, I finally understood what estrogen is all about. He speaks positively about hormone treatment in women after the menopause. He believes that, thanks to more thorough analyses and results, the view on estrogen is fortunately beginning to change. Naessén told me that several new studies show that estrogen has a strong protective effect against several illnesses, which means that it even decreases the risk of women dying during the treatment period compared to women given the placebo. For example, you can see that the risk of suffering heart and vascular problems is almost halved when undergoing hormone treatment.

Therefore, with Naessén's wise thoughts and explanations behind me, I feel that it's time to stick my neck out and once again say that estrogen is good for you. According to Naessén, there are clear signs that estrogen can decrease mortality by up to 30–40 percent during treatment, if you start treatment within 10 years of entering the menopause. This sounds amazing, but I was of course interested in his views of starting with estrogen as early as the perimenopause. The answer was as I thought. If you suffer from strong perimenopausal symptoms, you should consider hormone treatment, since it's the most effective and best-documented treatment according to Naessén. And his answer to the question of how long the treatment should be, was that it depends upon who you asked. If you asked him, the answer would be: »For as long as you need.«

This is completely revolutionary to me. More and more points to hormones being able to prolong life. Why doesn't the media write about this research that could influence women's lives for the better?

No more dangerous than other lifestyle factors

Despite the documented protective effects, there are disadvantages, as with all medical treatments. For example, I recently read an interesting summary in the Swedish book *Klimakteriet – en uppdatering* (»Menopause – an update«). It's intended, first and foremost, for primary care physicians and doctors in internal medicine, but also for gynecologists, nurses, midwives, and student doctors.

> »In summary, a combined estrogen and progesterone treatment (HRT) has been associated with a somewhat increased risk of breast cancer. The increased risk is of the same size as for many other lifestyle factors, such as delayed first pregnancy, and remains moderate even after long-term treatment.«

The words »as for many other lifestyle factors« stuck with me. They made me wonder if it would be better, for example, to stop eating red meat or to quit smoking, and take estrogen instead.

Maybe it can save
women from illness
and early death?
Is it something that,
in fact, is good for us?

Everything we do in life has advantages and disadvantages. All your choices affect how you feel and I believe there are other lifestyle factors more dangerous than estrogen. Just compare this to smoking – even if it makes you feel good at that moment, it's proven to be dangerous.

I believe we are unnecessarily frightened of estrogen. Think of it as a lifestyle factor and maybe the decision will be easier to take? Also remember that you have no idea of what the future holds. Who knows, I might get breast cancer in a couple of years or I may live to be 120. Or I might get run over by a car tomorrow? We know nothing. The only sure thing is that we will die one day or the other.

One very interesting thing is that, about 100 years ago, the average lifespan of women in Sweden was about 50 years. But once we started adding estrogen synthetically, the lifespan suddenly increased. These things may not be connected, but what if estrogen is a critical hormone that we, women, should not be without? Maybe it can save women from illness and early death? Is it something that, in fact, is good for us?

Generally, you could say that the criticism towards estrogen is diminishing. More and more gynecologists recommend taking estrogen supplements. I believe the attitude has changed partly because of the studies made after WHI, partly thanks to the advance of bioidentical estrogen in the hormone jungle. It is, after all, just like the body's own and therefore works well in our bodies. But despite bioidentical estrogen becoming more common, it's not something new. It came to Sweden as early as during the 70s but has not had its breakthrough until now.

Estrogen pioneer Mirjam Furuhjelm

There is a woman who, during her working life, was known as the estrogen pioneer. Her name was Mirjam Furuhjelm (1908–2003) and she was a pioneer within Swedish gynecology. As early as the end of the 1960s, she started recommending estrogen supplements according to her conviction that, as long as a woman is alive, she should make her life as good as possible. She, herself, started with estrogen in her 50s and lived to be 94.

Is estrogen dangerous?

In the book, largely about estrogen, Blod, svett och tårar (»Blood, sweat, and tears«), by the journalist Lena Katarina Swanberg, there is a wonderful passage where Mirjam Furuhjelm draws a parallel to diabetes:

> »Well, it's common sense. A person with diabetes needs additional insulin. She whose ovaries no longer work needs additional estrogen. And what's more, I would rather feel really well for five years than live ten years like a dog.«

On the question about what she thought about the movement recommending short-term treatment, she answered: »Do they believe the functioning of the ovaries will return afterwards?«

Swanberg's book was released in 2003 and was, deep down, very critical of estrogen. This was probably not the only book that criticized the hormone, bearing in mind that the WHI study changed the attitude of the entire world. But the interesting thing in this context, is that Furuhjelm was born in 1908 and, despite the WHI study, she stood her ground throughout her career, convinced that estrogen was something good. She also spoke widely about the importance of estrogen to our mental health. »It's idiotic that estrogen's advantages to mental health are not emphasized more in the debate,« she says in Swanberg's book.

And I am inclined to agree. Why doesn't anyone talk about how important estrogen is for making us feel less down, low, and depressed? Would it be the end for the advocates of anti-depressant medicines? Is that why no one dares? But it is indeed difficult to know which came first, the chicken or the egg. As I said before, I believe that lack of sleep is the root of all evil. Estrogen influences the sleep hormone positively and enables us to sleep and, when we sleep better, we start to feel better again.

I will end this chapter with yet another quote from estrogen pioneer Mirjam from Lena Katarina Swanberg's book:

> »If the body doesn't produce insulin, the illness is called diabetes. Without vitamin C, the body develops an illness called rickets. If a gland stops producing estrogen, the body begins its journey into senility. It's just as feasible that the gynecologist gives a middle-aged woman estrogen as it is for an optician to suggest reading glasses.«

If and when you take estrogen is entirely your own decision. The most important thing is that you have enough knowledge to make the right decision. Absorb information from different angles and don't trust blindly in what one person or another says. With sufficient knowledge, you will be able to choose whether to jump onto the hormone train or not. My hope is that what I have taught you might help you on your way. Don't forget that it is you who get to decide over your own body.

CHAPTER 12

Don't miss the progesterone

Do you remember me talking about the dance between hormones? That the hormones, just like the characters in *Dirty Dancing*, must be synchronized, otherwise nothing works? The hormonal worries we experience when they are a little at loggerheads isn't fun. I have also mentioned that estrogen can't be taken without progesterone. In this chapter I will talk about progesterone as a complement but also about a type of progesterone that may be taken on its own without estrogen.

Combining estrogen with progesterone

A synthetic form of progesterone, called progestin, is often found in the contraceptive pill. One of the side effects of the contraceptive pill is said to be melancholy, which can be traced to this particular intake of progestin. Therefore, many people choose to take the minipill instead, which contains a lower dose of progestin than the normal contraceptive pill.

During the perimenopause, the exact opposite is true. Symptoms such as sleeping problems and melancholy are not the result of having too much progesterone in your body, but rather *not having enough*. You could say that it is because of insufficient levels of progesterone that we feel worse, or

»I find hormones difficult. When I started with bioidentical progesterone cream, I started sleeping again, but my best friend did not feel well at all using it. What should I do?«

CAMILLA, 39

more accurately, because of an imbalance between estrogen and progesterone since it's the progesterone that starts to decrease first.

Now you may wonder why you can't add only additional progesterone if progesterone levels decrease before estrogen levels. For some reason, Swedish gynecologists normally only prescribe progesterone as a part of an HRT treatment. It's still a relatively unexplored area and, since there are no major studies to suggest that this would be enough to start with, it's not recommended today.

The tips I have given on how you can find a cure for your problems through lifestyle changes are especially useful when the hormonal imbalance is at an early stage. But when the lifestyle changes are not enough, it might be time to start thinking about estrogen and progesterone.

As I have mentioned earlier, they are both part of an HRT treatment. I have also mentioned that bioidentical estrogen is to be preferred over the synthetic. The same thing applies to progesterone.

Several studies confirm that bioidentical progesterone is preferred. As early as 2005, a French study of over 80,000 women showed clearly that the risk of breast cancer increased in the group taking synthetic progesterone, but no heightened risk was found in the patients given natural progesterone.

During the last few years, creams containing bioidentical progesterone have arrived on the market. They can be ordered online and have had a large and positive breakthrough, not least thanks to Mia Lundin, a Swedish midwife who lives in the US but also works in Sweden. Mia has made women feel better from bioidentical hormones, and recommends, among other things, progesterone cream. Progesterone cream isn't approved by FDA but is still considered an alternative method. Many women experience that it has helped them to sleep and calmed down the wound-up feeling in their bodies.

Despite Swedish gynecologists not always recommending it, today many women use the bioidentical progesterone cream before they start taking estrogen, in other words *not* as part of HRT. I have done this myself. The cream is applied where your skin is thin, I normally put it on the inside of my underarms or thighs. Dosage is difficult because how much to use is very individual.

When I started, I became incredibly calm and sleepy. For a long time, my body had felt hyper, the way you do when hormones start to become unbalanced. My gynecologist told me that my experience, on the whole, was similar to other people's descriptions. That you are feeling calm, the worry in your body disappears, and your sleep is improved. But she also told me that progesterone cream is a hot topic in her profession, since many patients use the cream without knowing what it does.

What gynecologists object to above all else is that there have been no studies that have shown that progesterone cream provides adequate protection to the endometrium, which means they will not recommend it as a progesterone complement in an HRT treatment.

After having made all the lifestyle changes I have described – taking melatonin, tried progesterone cream, and sometimes using Atarax – I had finally come to the point where it wasn't quite enough to rid me of my problems. I started approaching menopause. At that point, we agreed that I should stop everything (apart from the positive lifestyle changes) and *only* try estrogen.

As a progesterone complement to my estrogen treatment, I have chosen a hormone coil that works like a normal contraceptive but also releases progesterone locally which protects the endometrium. It is, however, a synthetic progesterone. I chose the coil since I am worried about feeling low (as many people are with the contraceptive pill). But if it's only released locally, the risk of side effects, such as feeling low, is minimal. If there was an alternative bioidentical progesterone in the form of a coil to protect the endometrium, I would choose that instead.

The advice isn't always unanimous

I can't stop wondering why gynecologists have such differences of opinion. For example, my sister-in-law's gynecologist considered progesterone cream to be an American PR stunt and that it should definitely not be used. The gynecologist of a close friend said that the notion of bioidentical progesterone being better than synthetic was nonsense – she meant that there were no grounds for such a claim. Ask your friends what their gynecologists say about progesterone and you will be surprised. Everyone says different things.

It was incredibly liberating when a gynecologist on prime-time TV admitted that not everyone in the business had the time to keep track of the latest research. In other words, maybe not all gynecologists know that hormone symptoms can be kept in check for a couple of years with only progesterone cream before the need to pull out the big HRT toolbox?

If you decide to take hormones and there are hormones available which are largely reminiscent of the body's own, I think that it must be better than taking synthetic equivalents. There are several studies that show how well the bioidentical progesterone interacts with the bioidentical estrogen and that this is the best combination for women, and with the least risk of side effects. Perhaps the medical profession should also take this on-board and not just the scientists? It may be new and modern, but everything points to this being what is best for us.

CHAPTER 13

Look outside yourself

I can see that the trend in the health business is aimed more and more towards »looking inwards.« How do *I* feel? What can *I* do to feel better? I completely agree. In order to understand yourself and find well-being in your own life, it's important to listen to yourself and to your body's signals. But I also think it's important to look outwards. I believe you should take yourself and your symptoms very seriously and try all the methods you can to feel better and find your perimenopower, but I also want you to take a look around. Is there anything outside of yourself that can make you feel better?

The value in sharing experiences

I am allergic to the kind of naval-gazing that's prevalent today and I am convinced that people need one another to feel better. That we can get more out of each other's experiences and knowledge than of trying to reinvent the wheel by just looking at ourselves as individuals. The solutions aren't always within yourself. I believe that we humans must help one another.

Is there anything apart from the advice I have given in this book that automatically makes you feel better? I think many people would answer that their relationship with family and friends is something that greatly effects their well-being. There is even research that shows that the greatest happiness is achieved by helping others. Martin Luther King said something that I often come back to and which I think fits into this context: »Life's most persistent and urgent question is, what are you doing for others?«

How can we help one another through this tough period in life? With a strong, steady base within yourself, closeness to other people, and a will to look outwards, you can get as far as you want. We humans are pack animals, we are not biologically constructed to live alone, and solutions to problems are often considerably easier to find when we help one another.

Help one another

Of course, it's important to look inwards and discover what is most suitable to you and not trust blindly in what someone else says (not even me). Look for the signals and instincts in your own body. But when you have done that, maybe you can help someone else, just by sharing how you feel. Maybe you will be surprised at what you find in other people's banks of experience.

Simply, start talking about this with your nearest and dearest. Imagine the strength you might find in comparing symptoms, laughing, crying, and realizing that life is actually pretty good if you share and dare to accept help. There is such value in having friendships and helping your friends – something that might even make you feel better than all the natural remedies, exercise sessions, and estrogen plasters in the whole world.

CHAPTER 14

Your new beginning

One of the most important things to me, now that you have almost finished the book, is that you realize you are not alone. Apart from your friends, most women you meet at work, on the bus, in the shop, at the gym also have problems at certain times of their lives. My intention with this book is to make you understand how your body works and that what you are experiencing isn't an illness, but a state.

Give your body the best preconditions during this period. Try to avoid sleeping pills and anti-depressants for as long as you can. If you get to the point where you must take them, do it for a while until it changes. I believe you can really benefit from acceptance. Don't fight it. Try to find solutions instead. We will always experience difficult and trying times throughout our lives and there is some truth in the saying: »it's not about what you have, but how you deal with it.«

But maybe we also need to be more grateful that we grow old at all. Some of us never will. Try to find an approach that makes you see your perimenopause and your symptoms more positively. You have a superpower within you which, now, is hidden by strange symptoms. Find yourself again, for behind all the difficulties is your perimenopower, I promise.

Approaching burnout or the menopause?

In the future, think about how you interpret studies and articles in the media. Just because a new study shows that evening primrose oil is effective against menopause problems, doesn't necessarily mean it will help you. Even I, who work in health and media, sometimes find it difficult to choose which studies to trust. But one of the guidelines I normally follow is that the more participants in the study, the better. A study of 200,000 women has a much better chance of being trustworthy than one of only 200.

Therefore, be critical when reading the evening papers or magazines when they say that: »a study shows …« Results and facts may have been angled or made to fit for the sake of the article, and they may also have been found in a minor study with just a few participants. Or maybe they have looked at just a few people in a faraway country with completely different diets and lifestyles than where you live. The same study may have shown a completely different result if it had been done during different conditions with other participants. Unfortunately, one can also be certain that for every study that proves one thing, there is another that proves the opposite. In other words, you should be careful with what you choose to believe in. Give it some extra thought and try to find similar articles from reputable sources that show similar results.

My conclusion, after studying this subject for many years,

Use critical thinking!

is that I believe that the health profession sometimes too easily gives a diagnosis of depression or exhaustion, prescribing anti-depressants or sleeping pills and sick leave. What if there is simply a hormonal problem in these women and, if these hormones could be sorted out, maybe the phenomena of exhaustion would not be so widespread? What if they are not approaching a burnout but are, instead, approaching menopause? I don't wish to belittle exhaustion diagnoses, but I believe some of these women would feel so much better if their hormones were rebalanced. I think the connection is greater than anyone realizes, and I also think this is what my next health book must be about.

Make sure you get the right help

I have learnt a great deal during my perimenopause and I have also learnt much while carrying out the research for this book. Above all, I have learnt not to be so quick to believe what other people say, even if they have the authority of a doctor or a health food advisor. I believe you gain more from being open to new knowledge and making your own decisions. You are, after all, the one who will have to live with the decision in the end.

Don't believe what the newspapers tell you, and take everything that you read on the internet with a pinch of salt. True or not, there are some strange studies out there. For example, I read about a Japanese survey showing that, if you do square dancing, your troubles will decrease. And don't believe that estrogen is dangerous, for there are just as many studies that show it to be vital.

If you go to your doctor and have a feeling you are not receiving the right kind of help, ask to be referred to a gynecologist. In my opinion, the doctor should refer you from the start. I had an interesting discussion with a close friend of mine who is a doctor at a local medical center about how he dealt with this type of problem. He could see a connection between hormonal problems and signing people off work sick. Today he refers his patients to a gynecologist, and the sick leave has decreased markedly. However, I do think this kind of action is rare.

Once you have been referred to a gynecologist, it's important that you feel comfortable with him or her. Should you feel misunderstood, you can hopefully change to another one.

Life is a gift. Seize every minute. It's not about *being given* help for your symptoms, it's about *going out and getting* help. Now that you know more about how your body works, you have the power. Don't sit and wait, instead go out and get help if you think that you need it. Finally, I would like to share a mantra that I like:

»This is the life you get. It's not a rehearsal.«

I try to live that way as much as I can. I try to be grateful and not become overwhelmed with things. I try to realize that I have a superpower and constantly remind myself of it. I often think about the singer Laleh who sings about how wonderful it is to have a moment on earth. I also think about how we shouldn't worry so much, that maybe we should be more relaxed about things. As far as I know, this is the only life we have. It's not a rehearsal. Try to make the best of it, even if things are sometimes going against you. Give yourself the best preconditions and you will see that everything will be OK.

»Whenever I feel bad,
I use that feeling to
motivate me to work harder.
I only allow myself
one day to feel sorry
for myself.
When I'm not feeling my
best I ask myself,
'What are you
gonna do about it?'
I use the negativity to fuel
the transformation into
a better me.«

BEYONCÉ

Thank you

Thank you for reading this book, it was written for you. If you would like to share your own experiences, there are many of us who would like to hear them. Please use the hashtag #perimenopower so that, together, we can make even more women understand that they are not alone in the chaos of the perimenopause. You can also follow mine and the book's journey on the Instagram account @perimenopower should you wish to know more, or just to say »hi«.

Thank you Ehrlin Publishing for believing in my idea. Thanks to Elin Westerberg, my editor, who has been a rock throughout this whole process. You have given me invaluable advice! Another person who has been invaluable is Doctor Evelina Idenfeldt. Without you there would never have been a book. I would also like to take the opportunity to thank the other doctors who have allowed me to interview them and also Doctor Margareta Nordenvall whom I, myself, have been seeing for several years.

Thank you Eva Lindeberg who has designed the book exactly how I wanted it.

Thanks to my sisters Monica and Anna who have supported me the entire way. Your support, when I have been struck by self-doubt, has meant so much. Thanks also to Tomas, for being there when I needed encouragement.

Thanks also to my fantastic friends – none mentioned, none forgotten. Thanks for putting up with me, for listening and believing in me and making me feel loved and appreciated.

I especially want to thank my sons, Ville and David, who have been forced to listen, for such a long time, to my long ramblings on a subject which isn't at the top of the list for teenage boys. Thank you for being there. You are the light in my life. I would be nothing without you.

And last, but not least. Thank you, Mum and Dad, for teaching me never to stop dreaming. That everything is possible as long as you want it deeply enough. I know you applaud me from Heaven, Dad.

Katarina Wilk

References

Allmen, Tara (2016). *Menopause Confidential*. New York: HarperOne.

Burke, Tina M., et al. (2015). Effects of caffeine on the human circadian clock in vivo and in vitro. *Science Translational Medicine*, 7(305). DOI:10.1126/SCITRANSLMED.AAC5125

Burkholder, Amy (2007, January 20). Perimenopause: Hormone ups and downs can last years. *CNN*. Retrieved from http://edition.cnn.com/2007/health/01/10/peri.menopause/

Davey, Gwyneth K., et al. (2003). EPIC-Oxford: lifestyle characteristics and nutrient intakes in a cohort of 33 883 meat-eaters and 31 546 non meat-eaters in the UK. *Public Health Nutrition*, 6(3), 259–269. DOI:10.1079/PHN2002430

Dolgen, Ellen (2014, December 22). A look at menopause through the ages. *Huffington Post*. Retrieved from https://www.huffingtonpost.com/ellen-sarver-dolgen/history-of-menopause_b_6159614.html

Eckerman, Ingrid (2017). Vad ska vi äta och varför. *AllmänMedicin, Tidskrift för svensk förening för allmänmedicin*, 3(38).

Ellenbogen, Jeffrey M. (2005). Cognitive benefits of sleep and their loss due to sleep deprivation. *Neurology*, 64(7). DOI:10.1212/01.WNL.0000164850.68115.81

Fryer, Bronwyn (2006, October). Sleep deficit: The performance killer. *Harvard Business Review*.

Gottfried, Sara (2015). *The Hormone Reset Diet*. New York: HarperOne.

Hammar, Mats, et al. (1990). Does physical exercise influence the frequency of postmenopausal hot flushes? *Acta Obstetricia et Gynecologica Scandinavica*, 69(5), 409–412. DOI:10.3109/00016349009013303

Harpaz, Mickey (2013, October 12). The history of menopause. *Menopause Matters*. Retrieved from http://menopausematterstoday.com/the-history-of-menopause/

Harvard Womens´s Health Watch (2018, August 24). *Perimenopause: Rocky road to menopause.* Retrieved from https://www.health.harvard.edu/ womens-health/perimenopause-rocky-road-to-menopause

Johansson, Martina (2017). *Hormonbibeln 2.0: För kvinnor genom hela livet.* Stockholm: Pagina.

Kim, Min-Ju, et al. (2014). Association between physical activity and menopausal symptoms in perimenopausal women. *BMC Womens Health, 14*(122). DOI:10.1186/1472-6874-14-122

Kirby, Julia (2013, May 13). Change the world and get to bed by 10:00. *Harvard Business Review.*

Le, Lap Tai, & Sabaté, Joan (2014). Beyond meatless, the health effects of vegan diets: Findings from the Adventist cohorts. *Nutrients, 6*(6), 2131–2147. DOI:10.3390/NU6062131

Lee, Duck-chuul, et al. (2014). Leisure-time running reduces all cause and cardiovascular mortality risk. *Journal of the American College of Cardiology, 64*(5), 472–481. DOI:10.1016/J.JACC.2014.04.058

Linde, Klaus, et al. (2008). St John's wort for major depression. *Cochrane Database of Systematic Reviews.* DOI:10.1002/14651858.CD000448.PUB3

Liu, Tong-Zu, et al. (2016). Sleep duration and risk of all-cause mortality: A flexible, non-linear, meta-regression of 40 prospective cohort studies. *Sleep Medicine Reviews, 32*, 28–36. DOI:10.1016/J. SMRV.2016.02.005

Lundin, Mia (2011). Kaos i kvinnohjärnan. *The Center for Hormonal and Nutritional Balance Inc.*

Lundin, Mia (2012, November 1). Samspelet mellan kvinnohormoner och signalsubstanser. *Kostrådgivarna.* Retrieved from http://www.kostradgi-varna.se/2012/11/samspelet-mellan-kvinnohormoner-och-signalsubstan-ser/

Makara-Studzinska, Marta, et al. (2014). Epidemiology of the symptoms of menopause – an intercontinental review. *Menopause Review/Przeglqd Menopauzalny*, 13(3), 203–211. DOI:10.5114/pm.2014.43827

Mandal, Ananya (2013, December 2). What are hormones? *News Medical Life Sciences*. Retrieved from https://www.news-medical.net/health/ What-are-Hormones.aspx

Manson, JoAnn E., et al. (2017). Menopausal hormone therapy and long-term all-cause and cause-specific mortality: The Women's Health Initiative randomized trials. *JAMA*, 318(10), 927–938. DOI:10.1001/ jama.2017.11217

Minkin, Mary Jane, & Wright, Carol V. (2005). *A Woman's Guide to Menopause and Perimenopause*. New Haven and London: Yale University Press.

Nayak, Gavathry, et al. (2014). Effect of yoga therapy on physical and psychological quality of life of perimenopausal women in selected coastal areas of Karnataka, India. *Journal of Mid-Life Health*, 5(4), 180–185. DOI:10.4103/0976-7800.145161

Somers, Suzanne (2013). *I'm Too Young for This!: The Natural Hormone Solution to Enjoy Perimenopause*. New York: Harmony Books.

Spetz Holm, Anna-Clara, et al. (2014). *Klimakteriet – en uppdatering*. Lund: Studentlitteratur.

Stenholtz, David (2017). Vegansk kost – många fördelar finns men kunskap krävs. AllmänMedicin, *Tidskrift för svensk förening för allmänmedicin*, 3(38).

Sternfeld, Barbara, & Dugan, Sheila (2001). Physical activity and health during the menopausal transition. *Obstetrics and Gynecology Clinics*, 38(3), 537–566. DOI:10.1016/j.ogc.2011.05.008

Swanberg, Lena Katarina (2003). *Blod, svett och tårar: En ilsken bok om östrogen*. Stockholm: Bokförlaget DN.

Interviews

Evelina Sande Idenfeldt, Chief Physician of obstetrics and gynecology. Continuous phone interviews, 2017, September through 2018, February.

Mats Hammar, Professor Emeritus of obstetrics and gynecology at Linköping University. Email interview, 2017, November.

Torbjörn Åkerstedt, Professor of psychology at Karolinska Institutet. Email interview, 2018, January.

Tord Naéssen, Professor of obstetrics and gynecology at Uppsala University. Phone interview, 2018, January.

Useful web sites:

www.menopause.org
www.whi.org
www.imsociety.org